Differential Diagnosis in Small Animal Medicine

T0258396

Differential Diagnosis in Small Animal Medicine

Second Edition

By

Alex Gough
MA VetMB CertSAM CertVC PGCert MRCVS

Kate Murphy
BVSc (Hons) DSAM DipECVIM-CA MRCVS PGCert (HE)

WILEY Blackwell

This edition first published 2015 © 2015 by John Wiley & Sons, Ltd

Registered Office
John Wiley & Sons, Ltd, The Atrium, Southern Gate, Chichester, West Sussex, PO19 8SQ, UK

Editorial Offices
9600 Garsington Road, Oxford, OX4 2DQ, UK
The Atrium, Southern Gate, Chichester, West Sussex, PO19 8SQ, UK
1606 Golden Aspen Drive, Suites 103 and 104, Ames, Iowa 50010, USA

For details of our global editorial offices, for customer services and for information about how to apply for permission to reuse the copyright material in this book please see our website at www.wiley.com/wiley-blackwell

The right of the author to be identified as the author of this work has been asserted in accordance with the UK Copyright, Designs and Patents Act 1988.

Designations used by companies to distinguish their products are often claimed as trademarks. All brand names and product names used in this book are trade names, service marks, trademarks or registered trademarks of their respective owners. The publisher is not associated with any product or vendor mentioned in this book. It is sold on the understanding that the publisher is not engaged in rendering professional services. If professional advice or other expert assistance is required, the services of a competent professional should be sought.

The contents of this work are intended to further general scientific research, understanding, and discussion only and are not intended and should not be relied upon as recommending or promoting a specific method, diagnosis, or treatment by health science practitioners for any particular patient. The publisher and the author make no representations or warranties with respect to the accuracy or completeness of the contents of this work and specifically disclaim all warranties, including without limitation any implied warranties of fitness for a particular purpose. In view of ongoing research, equipment modifications, changes in governmental regulations, and the constant flow of information relating to the use of medicines, equipment, and devices, the reader is urged to review and evaluate the information provided in the package insert or instructions for each medicine, equipment, or device for, among other things, any changes in the instructions or indication of usage and for added warnings and precautions. Readers should consult with a specialist where appropriate. The fact that an organization or Website is referred to in this work as a citation and/or a potential source of further information does not mean that the author or the publisher endorses the information the organization or Website may provide or recommendations it may make. Further, readers should be aware that Internet Websites listed in this work may have changed or disappeared between when this work was written and when it is read. No warranty may be created or extended by any promotional statements for this work. Neither the publisher nor the author shall be liable for any damages arising herefrom.

Library of Congress Cataloging-in-Publication Data

Gough, Alex, author.
 Differential diagnosis in small animal medicine / by Alex Gough, Kate Murphy. – Second edition.
  pages ; cm
 Includes bibliographical references and index.
 ISBN 978-1-118-40968-8 (pbk.)
1. Dogs–Diseases–Diagnosis–Handbooks, manuals, etc. 2. Cats–Diseases–Diagnosis–Handbooks, manuals, etc.
3. Diagnosis, Differential–Handbooks, manuals, etc. I. Murphy, K. F. (Kate F.), author. II. Title.
 [DNLM: 1. Animal Diseases–diagnosis–Handbooks. 2. Diagnosis, Differential–Handbooks.
3. Veterinary Medicine–methods–Handbooks. SF 748]
 SF991.G672 2015
 636.089'6075–dc23

                                                         2014034803

A catalogue record for this book is available from the British Library.

Wiley also publishes its books in a variety of electronic formats. Some content that appears in print may not be available in electronic books.

Cover image: dog and cat – iStockphoto © tetsuomorita; all other images – reproduced with permission of the University of Bristol Photographic Unit

Set in 9/10.5pt Sabon by SPi Publisher Services, Pondicherry, India
Printed and bound by CPI Group (UK) Ltd, Croydon, CR0 4YY

C9781118409688_081123

Contents

Introduction

The first edition of this book was written by Alex Gough to fill a gap in the market. The aim was to provide a ready list of differential diagnoses to assist in the investigation of challenging medical cases, and the sales of the book would suggest this was a success.

This second edition has been co-authored by Alex Gough and Kate Murphy. Content has been reviewed and expanded where needed and some sections have been removed.

This book provides a ready reference for differential diagnoses for the majority of medical presentations that are encountered in general practice, including both common and uncommon conditions. This text should be of use to veterinary students, general practitioners, veterinary interns, residents and anyone who cannot fully carry these lists around in their heads. We hope clinicians find it useful.

The differential diagnosis list is one of the most important aspects of the problem-oriented approach to clinical diagnosis. For those who are not familiar with the problem-oriented approach, a brief outline follows.

As the name implies, problem-oriented medical management (POMM) concentrates on the individual problems of a patient. A differential diagnosis list should be made for each and every problem that is found in a patient, whether in the history, the physical examination, imaging or clinicopathological tests. Although superficially this may not sound very 'holistic', in fact, if all the patient's problems are considered individually, the whole patient will have been evaluated, without falling into the trap of presuming that all of the findings are caused by a single condition. Some problems are of course less specific and less emphasis is given to the problem solving on those signs, e.g. lethargy and inappetence in a vomiting, jaundiced pet.

Differential Diagnosis in Small Animal Medicine, Second Edition.
Alex Gough and Kate Murphy.
© 2015 John Wiley & Sons, Ltd. Published 2015 by John Wiley & Sons, Ltd.

The problem-oriented approach starts with a thorough history, and it is important to discover what the owners perceive to be the main problems – after all, they usually know their animal better than the clinician does. However, there may be relevant historical signs that the owners had not considered significant, so failing to systematically ask all the questions which could be of importance in a case can lead to overlooking important information.

In every case, a complete physical examination should be carried out, including body systems that are not apparently of immediate concern.

Once the history has been taken and the physical examination has been completed, the clinician should list every problem (ideally rank the problems) that has been discovered. Problems may include such findings as exercise intolerance, pruritus, pyrexia or a heart murmur. A differential diagnosis list should then be created for every problem. The list should be appropriate to that animal. There is no point listing feline leukaemia virus as a likely diagnosis in a dog!

An attempt should also be made to categorise the conditions in order of likelihood, or at least into common and uncommon. Although the more common conditions have been indicated in this book with an asterisk (*), there are few objective data regarding the true incidence of conditions, and the estimate of incidence is largely subjective and influenced by the authors' geographical location and caseload. Familiarity with how common conditions are and their local incidence will help prioritise differential lists. The clinician can then select diagnostic tests in a rough order of probability, although rarer but life-threatening conditions, such as hypoadrenocorticism, should also be ruled out early in the course of investigations. Some authorities rightly point out that emphasis should be placed on historical and physical signs and that 'over-investigating' can be expensive and potentially detrimental to the patient.

However, it is possible to place too much importance on probabilities and how commonly a condition occurs. The newly qualified veterinary surgeon will often look for the rare but exciting and memorable condition they learned about at college, while the experienced practitioner will often remind them that 'common things are common' and suggest they restrict their investigations only to commonly encountered conditions. The ideal approach is probably somewhere in between. The problem-oriented approach means that all differentials should have been considered and investigations can be targeted, but if a diagnosis is not made, the list should be revisited to consider other appropriate testing

Some authorities prefer to categorise the initial approach to a case differently and describe the subjective and objective assessment of a patient as part of the SOAP approach (Subjective, Objective, Assessment, Plan). The principle is the same however, in that a detailed history or physical examination is the basis of the initial differential list.

Once the differential diagnosis list has been formulated, the clinician is in a position to select appropriate tests to aid in making a definitive diagnosis. Prioritising the selection of diagnostic tests helps avoid placing undue financial strain on the client and inappropriate or unnecessary testing on the patient. Tests may be prioritised on such factors as the number of conditions which will be ruled in and out, the sensitivity and specificity of the tests; the risk/benefit to the patient ratio; the financial cost/benefit to the client ratio; the incidence or prevalence of the condition being tested for and the importance of the condition being tested for (e.g. hypoadrenocorticism is uncommon, but the consequences of failing to diagnose it may be serious).

After the results of initial testing have been obtained the clinician may be in a position to make a definitive diagnosis. Often, however, it is necessary to refine the differential list and select further appropriate testing. The differential list may be reformulated as often as is necessary until a diagnosis for that problem is made. Often, a single diagnosis will tie in all the problems satisfactorily. However, in many cases, particularly in geriatric patients, concurrent disorders will require multiple diagnoses.

For problem cases in which a clear diagnosis is not made or the patient fails to respond to treatment as expected, returning to the beginning with the history and physical examination, with the condition often having progressed, can be helpful. However, very few tests are 100% sensitive and specific, and many 'definitive' diagnoses in fact leave room for some doubt. The clinician should never be afraid to revise the initial diagnosis if further evidence comes to light. Those who are concerned that failing to make the correct diagnosis in every case is somehow a sign of inferior clinical abilities should take heart from a 2004 study from the School of Veterinary Medicine at the University of California. In this paper, clinical and post-mortem diagnoses of 623 dogs treated between 1989 and 1999 at the Veterinary Teaching Hospital were compared. It was found that the post-mortem diagnosis, presumed to be the correct diagnosis, differed from the clinical diagnosis in approximately one-third of cases.

This book is organised into five parts. Part 1 deals with signs likely to be uncovered during history taking. Part 2 deals with signs encountered at the physical examination. Part 3 deals with imaging findings, Part 4 with clinicopathological findings and Part 5 with electrophysiological findings.

The individual lists are largely organised alphabetically. The more common conditions are labelled with an asterisk, but, as stated above, whether a condition is considered to be common is largely a matter of subjective opinion. Those conditions that are predominantly or exclusively found only in dogs are marked with a (D) and those in cats are marked with a (C).

Sources for the information in this book are wide ranging. A large number of textbooks, were consulted, but in most cases it was necessary to expand the lists found in these sources, using information from veterinary journals and conference proceedings.

Although there are undoubtedly omissions from some of the lists, encompassing as this book does virtually the whole of small animal veterinary medicine, we have tried to make it as comprehensive as possible. We would be happy to hear of any omissions, corrections or comments on the text, which can be e-mailed with any supporting references to alex.gough@bathvetreferrals.co.uk.

The following colleagues provided comments on the text of the first edition for which we are grateful: Simon Platt BVM&S DipACVIM DipECVN MRCVS, Chris Belford BVSc DVSc FACVSc RCVS Specialist Pathologist Dip Wldl Mgt, Theresa McCann BVSc CertSAM MRCVS, Rosie McGregor BVSc CertVD CertVC MRCVS, Mark Bush MA VetMB CertSAS MRCVS, Alison Thomas BVSc CertSAM MRCVS, Mark Maltman BVSc CertSAM CertVC MRCVS, Panagiotis Mantis DVM DipECVDI MRCVS, Axiom Laboratories, Stuart Caton BA VetMB CertSAM MRCVS, Tim Knott BSc BVSc CertVetOphth MRCVS, Lisa Phillips CertVR BVetMed MRCVS, Roderick MacGregor BVM&S CertVetOphth CertSAS MRCVS and Mark Owen BVSc CertSAO MRCVS. Any errors are of course ours and not theirs. We are also grateful to Justinia Wood at Wiley for her support in this project.

Key

* = more common condition
(D) = condition seen exclusively or predominantly in dogs
(C) = condition seen exclusively or predominantly in cats
q.v. = more information can be found on this condition elsewhere in this book – see Index

PART 1
HISTORICAL SIGNS

1.1 General, systemic and metabolic historical signs

1.1.1 Polyuria/polydipsia

Diet
Increased salt intake
Very-low-protein diet

Drugs/toxins
Aminophylline
Corticosteroids
Delmadinone acetate
Diuretics
Ethylene glycol
Indomethacin
 • Lilies
Lithium
 • Melamine
NPK fertilisers
Paraquat
Phenobarbitone
Potassium bromide

Differential Diagnosis in Small Animal Medicine, Second Edition.
Alex Gough and Kate Murphy.
© 2015 John Wiley & Sons, Ltd. Published 2015 by John Wiley & Sons, Ltd.

Primidone
Proligestone
* Raisins/grapes
Terfenadine
Theophylline
Vitamin D rodenticides

Electrolyte disorders

Hypercalcaemia *q.v.*
Hypernatraemia *q.v.*
* Primary
* Secondary to dehydration, lack of intake, excessive loss of water, severe vomiting/diarrhoea, etc.

Hypokalaemia *q.v.*

Endocrine disease

Acromegaly
Diabetes mellitus*
Diabetes insipidus
* Central
* Nephrogenic

Hyperadrenocorticism
Hyperthyroidism* (C)
Hypoadrenocorticism (D)
Insulinoma
Pheochromocytoma
Primary hyperaldosteronism
Primary hyperparathyroidism

Hepatobiliary disease, e.g.

Hepatic neoplasia* *q.v.*
Hepatitis/cholangiohepatitis* *q.v.*

Infectious disease, e.g.

Toxaemia, e.g.
* Pyometra*

Miscellaneous

Congenital lack of ADH receptors
Hypothalamic disease
Pericardial effusion

Polycythaemia
Psychogenic*

Neoplasia*

Physiological
Exercise
High environmental temperature

Renal disorders
Acute kidney injury* *q.v.*
Chronic kidney disease* *q.v.*
Following urethral obstruction*
Glomerulonephritis
Primary renal glycosuria
Pyelonephritis
Renal medullary washout

Note: Polyuria and polydipsia are considered together here, since one will lead to the other, with only a few exceptions. These include polydipsia in the face of obstructive lower urinary tract disease or oliguric renal failure and polyuria which is not matched by fluid intake, in which case dehydration will rapidly follow. None of these scenarios are encountered commonly in practice. Polydipsia without polyuria can occur in situations of increased urinary loss of fluid, such as after strenuous exercise.

1.1.2 Weight loss

Decreased nutrient intake
Anorexia* *q.v.*
Diet
  • Poor-quality diet
  • Underfeeding
Dysphagia *q.v.*
Oral disease, e.g.
  • Dental disease
  • Masticatory myositis
  • Temporomandibular joint disease
Regurgitation *q.v.*

Increased nutrient loss

Burns
Chronic blood loss
- Epistaxis *q.v.*
- Haematemesis *q.v.*
- Haematuria *q.v.*
- Melaena *q.v.*

Diabetes mellitus/diabetic ketoacidosis*
Effusions *q.v.*
Fanconi syndrome (D)
Intestinal parasites*
Neoplasia*
Protein-losing enteropathy*
Protein-losing nephropathy

Increased nutrient use

Endocrine, e.g.
Hyperthyroidism* (C)

Neoplasia*

Physiological
Cold environment
Exercise
Fever *q.v.*
Lactation*
Pregnancy*

Maldigestion/malabsorption

Cardiac failure
Exocrine pancreatic insufficiency
Hepatic failure/bile salt deficiency *q.v.*
Hypoadrenocorticism (D)
Neoplasia*
Renal disease* *q.v.*
Small intestinal disease* *q.v.*, e.g.
- Antibiotic-responsive diarrhoea
- Inflammatory bowel disease
- Lymphangiectasia

Regurgitation and vomiting* q.v.

1.1.3 Weight gain

Decreased energy utilisation, e.g.
- Decreased exercise

Fluid accumulation

Ascites* *q.v.*
Peripheral oedema *q.v.*
Pleural effusion

Increased body fat

Overeating
Boredom
Excessive appetite (normal in some breeds)
High-calorie diets
Overfeeding*

Endocrinopathies
Acromegaly
Hyperadrenocorticism
Hypogonadism
Hypothyroidism* (D)
Insulinoma

Increased organ size

Hepatomegaly* *q.v.*
Renomegaly *q.v.*
Splenomegaly* *q.v.*
Uterine enlargement *q.v.*
- Pregnancy*
- Pyometra*

Neoplasia

Large abdominal mass (often associated with poor body condition)*
Drugs, e.g.
- Corticosteroids

1.1.4 Polyphagia

Behavioural/psychological
Boredom
Normal in some breeds*
Psychogenic, e.g. problem with satiety centre

Diet
Highly palatable food*
Poor-quality food

Drugs, e.g.
Benzodiazepines
Corticosteroids
Mirtazapine
Progestagens

Endocrine
Acromegaly
Diabetes mellitus*
Hyperadrenocorticism
Hyperthyroidism *(C)
Insulinoma

Increased nutrient loss, e.g.
Exocrine pancreatic insufficiency
Malabsorption
  • Small intestinal disease

Increased nutrient use, e.g.
Neoplasia

Malassimilation q.v.

Physiological
Cold environment
Increased exercise
Lactation
Pregnancy

1.1.5 Anorexia/inappetence

Anorexia, primary

Intracranial disease, e.g.
- Hypothalamic neoplasia

Anorexia, secondary

Anosmia
- Chronic rhinitis *q.v.*
- Nasal neoplasia
- Other nasal disease
- Neurological disease

Endocrine disease, e.g.
- Diabetic ketoacidosis
- Hypoadrenocorticism (D)

Fever* *q.v.*

Gastrointestinal disease *q.v.*, e.g.
- Gastritis
- Inflammatory bowel disease*

Heart disease, e.g.
- Cardiac failure*

Hepatic disease* *q.v.*

Infection*

Metabolic abnormalities, e.g.
- Hypercalcaemia *q.v.*
- Hypokalaemia *q.v.*

Pain*

Pancreatic disease*, e.g.
- Pancreatitis

Renal disease* *q.v.*

Respiratory disease, e.g.
- Airway disease* *q.v.*
- Diaphragmatic hernia
- Pleural effusion* *q.v.*
- Pneumonia *q.v.*

Diet

Recent dietary changes*
Unpalatable diet*

Difficulty with mastication

Dental disease*
Lingual disease
Oral neoplasia*
Oral ulceration, e.g.
- Ingestion of caustic or acidic substances*
- Renal disease

Difficulty with prehension

Blindness *q.v.*
Myopathy, e.g.
- Masticatory myositis
- Tetanus

Pain on opening jaw, e.g.
- Mandibular or maxillary fracture
- Retrobulbar abscess
- Skull fractures
- Soft tissue trauma
- Temporomandibular joint disease

Trigeminal nerve disease, e.g.
- Neoplasia
- Trigeminal neuritis

Difficulty with swallowing

Pharyngeal disease
Foreign body*
Neoplasia
Neurological disease
Ulceration

Oesophageal disease, e.g.
Foreign body*
Megaoesophagus
Neoplasia
Stricture
Ulceration
Vascular ring anomaly

Drugs
- Acetazolamide
- Amiodarone
- Amphotericin B
- Bethanechol
- Bromocriptine
- Butorphanol
- Cardiac glycosides
- Chlorambucil
- Diazoxide
- Doxorubicin
- Fentanyl
- Hydralazine
- Itraconazole
- Ketoconazole
- Melphalan
- Methimazole
- Mitotane
- Nicotinamide
- Oxytetracycline (C)
- Penicillamine
- Theophylline
- Trimethoprim/sulphonamide (C)

Psychological/behavioural* factors
Altered schedule
New family members
New house
New pets

1.1.6   Failure to grow

With good body condition
Chondrodystrophy (normal in many breeds)* (D)
Endocrine disorders
- Congenital hyposomatotropism
  (pituitary dwarfism)
- Congenital hypothyroidism

With poor body condition

Dietary intolerance
Exocrine pancreatic insufficiency*
Inadequate nutrient intake
- Anorexia *q.v.*
- Poor-quality diet
- Underfeeding

Cardiac disorders, e.g.
- Congenital
- Endocarditis

Endocrine disease
- Diabetes insipidus
- Diabetes mellitus*
- Hypoadrenocorticism (D)

Gastrointestinal disease, e.g.
- Histoplasmosis
- Obstruction, e.g.
  - Foreign body*
  - Intussusception*
- Parasites*

Hepatic disorders, e.g.
- Hepatitis *q.v.*
- Portosystemic shunt

Inflammatory disease
Oesophageal disorders, e.g.
- Megaoesophagus *q.v.*
- Vascular ring anomaly (e.g. persistent right aortic arch)

Renal disease
- Congenital kidney disease
- Glomerulonephritis
- Pyelonephritis

1.1.7   Syncope/collapse

Cardiovascular dysfunction

Bradyarrhythmias q.v., e.g.
- High-grade second-degree heart block
- Sick sinus syndrome (D)

- Third-degree heart block

Myocardial failure

Myocardial infarction

Cardiac disease

- Congenital, e.g.
  - Aortic stenosis (D)
  - Pulmonic stenosis (D)
- Hypertrophic obstructive cardiomyopathy
- Pericardial effusion* (D)
- Pulmonary hypertension
- Arterial obstruction, e.g.
  - Neoplasia
  - Thrombosis

Shock *q.v.*

Tachyarrhythmias q.v.

- Supraventricular tachycardia*
- Ventricular tachycardia*

Drugs

Anti-arrhythmics, e.g.

- Atenolol
- Digoxin
- Propranolol
- Quinidine

Sedatives, e.g.

- Phenothiazines

Vasodilators, e.g.

- ACE inhibitors
- Hydralazine
- Nitroglycerine

Hypoxaemic disease

Carboxyhaemoglobinaemia

Methaemoglobinaemia

Pleural/thoracic disorders, e.g.

- Pleural effusion
- Pneumothorax
- Rib fractures

Respiratory disease

- Lower airway, e.g.
  - Pneumonia
  - Small airway disease
- Upper airway, e.g.
  - Brachycephalic obstructive airway syndrome
  - Laryngeal paralysis
  - Tracheal collapse
  - Tracheal obstruction
- Ventilation–perfusion mismatch, e.g.
  - Pulmonary thromboembolism (PTE)
  - Lung collapse

Right-to-left cardiac shunt, e.g.
- Reverse-shunting patent ductus arteriosus
- Severe anaemia

Metabolic/endocrine disorders

Diabetic ketoacidosis
Hypercalcaemia/hypocalcaemia *q.v.*
Hypernatraemia/hyponatraemia *q.v.*
Hyperthermia/hypothermia *q.v.*
Hypoglycaemia *q.v.*
Hyperkalaemia/hypokalaemia *q.v.*
Severe acidosis *q.v.*
Severe alkalosis *q.v.*
Pheochromocytoma
Hypoadrenocorticism
Insulinoma

Miscellaneous

Carotid sinus stimulation, e.g.
- Neoplasia
- Tight collar

Hyperventilation
Postural hypotension
Tussive/cough syncope

Myopathies

Corticosteroid myopathy
Exertional myopathy
Hypocalcaemic myopathy

Hypokalaemic myopathy
Malignant hyperthermia
Mitochondrial myopathy
Muscular dystrophy
Polymyopathy
Polymyositis
Protozoal myopathy

Neurological dysfunction

Brainstem disease
Diffuse cerebral dysfunction, e.g.
- Encephalopathy
- Haemorrhage
- Hydrocephalus
- Inflammation
- Oedema
- Space-occupying lesion
- Trauma

Fibrocartilaginous embolism
Glossopharyngeal neuralgia
Lower motor neurone disorders
- Endocrine neuropathies, e.g.
  - Diabetes mellitus*
  - Hyperadrenocorticism
  - Hypothyroidism* (D)
- Lumbosacral disease
- Paraneoplastic neuropathies, e.g.
  - Insulinoma
- Peripheral nerve neoplasia
- Polyneuropathy, e. g.
  - Polyradiculoneuropathy

Micturition-related collapse
Narcolepsy/cataplexy
Neuromuscular junction disorders
- Botulism
- Myasthenia gravis

Seizures *q.v.*
Swallowing-related collapse
Upper motor neurone disorders
- Central vestibular disease

- Cerebellar disease
- Cerebral disease
- Peripheral vestibular disease
- Spinal disease

Skeletal/joint disorders

Bilateral cranial cruciate disease
Bilateral hip disease
Discospondylitis
Intervertebral disc disease
Multiple myeloma
Osteoarthritis
Panosteitis
Patellar luxation
Polyarthritis

1.1.8 Weakness

Cardiovascular diseases

Bradyarrhythmias *q.v.*, e.g.
- High-grade second-degree heart block
- Sick sinus syndrome (D)
- Third-degree heart block

Congestive heart failure*
Hypertension* *q.v.*
Hypotension* *q.v.*
Pericardial effusion* *q.v.*
Tachyarrhythmias *q.v.*, e.g.
Ventricular tachycardia*
- Supraventricular tachycardia

Drugs/toxins

Alphachloralose
Anticoagulant rodenticides
Anticonvulsants
Antihistamines
Blue-green algae
Cannabis
Diclofenac sodium

Glucocorticoids
Hypotensive agents, e.g.
- Beta blockers
- Vasodilators

Ibuprofen
Insulin overdosage
Iron salts
Mistletoe
Opioids
Organophosphates
Petroleum distillates
Phenoxy acid herbicides
Pyrethrin/pyrethroids
Rhododendron
Salbutamol
Sedatives

Endocrine diseases

Diabetes mellitus*
Hyperadrenocorticism
Hyperparathyroidism
Hypoadrenocorticism (D)
Hypoparathyroidism
Hypothyroidism* (D)
Insulinoma

Haematological diseases

Anaemia* *q.v.*
Hyperviscosity syndrome, e.g. polycythaemia

Inflammatory/Immune-mediated diseases

Chronic inflammatory conditions*
Immune-mediated haemolytic anaemia* *q.v.*
Immune-mediated polyarthritis

Infectious diseases*

Bacterial
Viral
Fungal
Rickettsial
Protozoal and other parasitic diseases

Metabolic disease

Acid–base disorders
- Acidosis *q.v.*
- Alkalosis *q.v.*

Electrolyte disorders*
- Hypercalcaemia*/hypocalcaemia *q.v.*
- Hyperkalaemia/hypokalaemia* *q.v.*
- Hypernatraemia/hyponatraemia *q.v.*

Hepatic failure* *q.v.*

Hyper-/hypoglycaemia *q.v.*

Renal disease* *q.v.*

Neurological diseases

Intracranial disease, e.g.

Cerebrovascular accident
- Epilepsy* *q.v.*

Infection

Inflammation

Space-occupying lesions

Vestibular disease

Neuromuscular disease, e.g.
- Botulism
- Myasthenia gravis
- Myopathies
- Tick paralysis

Peripheral polyneuropathies

Drugs/toxins, e.g.
- Cisplatin
- Lead
- Vincristine

Endocrine disorders, e.g.
- Diabetes mellitus*
- Hyperadrenocorticism
- Hypothyroidism* (D)

Polyradiculoneuritis

Paraneoplastic disorders

Spinal cord disease q.v., e.g.

Fibrocartilaginous embolism

Infection
Inflammation
Intervertebral disc disease* (D)
Neoplasia
Trauma*

Vestibular disease q.v.
- Central vestibular disease
- Peripheral vestibular disease

Nutritional disorders

Cachexia, e.g.
Heart failure*
Neoplasia*

Inadequate calorie intake, e.g.
Anorexia* *q.v.*
Poor-quality diet

Specific nutrient deficiencies, e.g.
Minerals
Vitamins

Physiological factors

Over-exercise
Pain*
Stress/anxiety*

Respiratory diseases

Airway obstruction, e.g.
- Feline asthma* (C)
- Foreign body*
- Neoplasia *
- Pleural effusion*
- Pulmonary hypertension
- Pulmonary oedema* *q.v.*
- Pulmonary thromboembolism
Severe pulmonary parenchymal disease

Systemic disorders

Dehydration*
Fever* *q.v.*
Neoplasia*

1.2 Gastrointestinal/abdominal historical signs

1.2.1 Ptyalism/salivation/hypersalivation

Drugs/toxins

Adder bites
Alphachloralose
Baclofen
Batteries
Benzodiazepines
Bethanechol
Blue-green algae
Cannabis
Carbamate
Chocolate/theobromine
Cotoneaster
Cyanoacrylate adhesives
Daffodil
Dieffenbachia
Dinoprost tromethamine
Glyphosphate
Horse chestnut
Ivermectin
Ketamine
Laburnum
Levamisole (C)
Loperamide
Metronidazole
Mistletoe
NPK fertilisers
Organophosphates
Paracetamol
Paraquat
Phenoxy acid herbicides
Plastic explosives
Plants
Pyrethrin/pyrethroids

Pyridostigmine
Rhododendron
Rowan
Terfenadine
Toads
Trimethoprim/sulphonamide (C)
Xylazine

Nausea/regurgitation/vomiting q.v.*

Neurological disease
Cataplexy/narcolepsy
Hepatic encephalopathy
Intracranial neoplasia
Partial seizures

Normal breed variation, e.g.*
St Bernard

Oral cavity disease
Dental disease*
Foreign body*
Neoplasia*, e.g. tonsillar
Inability to close mouth, e.g.
  • Mandibular trauma*
  • Trigeminal nerve disease, e.g.
    Idiopathic trigeminal neuritis
    Infiltrating neoplasia, e.g.
    Lymphoma
    Nerve sheath tumours
Infection, e.g.
  • Rabies
Inflammation, e.g.
  • Faucitis*
  • Lip fold dermatitis
  • Gingivitis*
  • Glossitis*
  • Oesophagitis*
  • Stomatitis*

Ulceration*, e.g.
- Chronic kidney disease*
- Immune-mediated disease
- Ingestion of irritant substance

Physiological factors

Appetite stimulation*
Fear*
Stress*

Salivary gland disease q.v.

Salivary gland necrosis/sialadenitis
Salivary mucocoele
Sialadenosis

1.2.2 Gagging/retching

Congenital disease

Achalasia, e.g.
- Cricopharyngeal achalasia (D)

Cleft palate
Hydrocephalus

Inflammatory and infectious disease

Asthma* (C)
Bacterial encephalitis
Fungal disease
- Granuloma complex

Idiopathic glossopharyngitis
Laryngitis*
Nasopharyngeal disease, e.g. polyps (C)
Pharyngitis*
Rabies
Rhinitis*
Sialadenitis
Viral encephalitis

Neoplasia
Central nervous system
Epiglottis
Inner ear
Nasal
Pharyngeal
Tonsillar

Neurological disease
Brainstem disease
Cranial nerve defects (V, VII, IX, XII)
Encephalitis
Laryngeal paralysis*
Muscular dystrophy
Myasthenia gravis

Nutrition
Food texture and size

Respiratory disease (expectoration), e.g.
Bronchitis*
Haemorrhage
Pulmonary oedema*

Systemic disorders
Hypocalcaemia
Renal disease*

Toxic
Botulism
Ingestion of irritant chemical
Smoke

Trauma
Foreign body*
Pharyngeal haematoma
Styloid apparatus trauma
Tracheal rupture

1.2.3 Dysphagia

Infectious/inflammatory disease

Oral disease
Dental disease*
Osteomyelitis of the jaw
Periodontitis*
Pharyngitis*
Rabies
Retrobulbar abscess
Severe gingivitis*
Salivary gland disease, e.g.
- Sialadenitis

Tooth root abscess*
Ulceration, e.g.
- Ingestion of irritant substance
- Renal disease*

Neurological/neuromuscular disease

Cricopharyngeal achalasia
Myasthenia gravis
Myopathy, e.g.
- Masticatory myopathy

Trigeminal nerve disease, e.g.
- Intracranial disease
- Trigeminal neuritis

Obstruction

Foreign body*
Granuloma
Neoplasia
Sialocoele

Temporomandibular joint disease

Trauma
Fracture
Haematoma
Laceration

1.2.4 Regurgitation

Endocrine disease
Hypoadrenocorticism (D)
Hypothyroidism* (D)

Gastric disease (can develop regurgitation secondary to outflow obstruction)
Gastric dilatation/volvulus* (D)
Hiatal hernia
- Gastro-oeosophageal intussusception
Pyloric outflow obstruction, e.g.
- Foreign body*
- Neoplasia
- Pyloric stenosis

Immune-mediated disease
Dermatomyositis (D)
Polymyositis
Systemic lupus erythematosus

Neurological disease
Central nervous system disease, e.g.
Brainstem disease
Distemper infection (D)
Infection
Inflammation
Intracranial space-occupying lesion
Storage diseases
Trauma

Neuromuscular junctionopathies, e.g.
Anticholinesterase toxicity
Botulism
Myasthenia gravis
Tetanus

Peripheral neuropathies, e.g.
Giant cell axonal neuropathy (D)
Lead poisoning

Polyneuritis
Polyradiculoneuritis
- Idiopathic
- Tick paralysis

Oesophageal disease
Foreign body*
Granuloma, e.g. *Spirocerca lupi*
Mediastinal mass (extraluminal obstruction)
Megaoesophagus
- Idiopathic
- Acquired

Neoplasia
Oesophageal diverticulum
Oesophageal fistula
Oesophageal inclusion cysts
Oesophagitis*, e.g.
- Secondary to gastric reflux
- Severe vomiting
  - Post anaesthesia
  - Idiopathic
  - Ingestion irritants

Stricture
Vascular ring anomaly, e.g.
- Persistent right aortic arch

Salivary gland disease
Sialadenitis
Sialadenosis

1.2.5   Vomiting

ACUTE VOMITING

Dietary
Dietary indiscretion*
Dietary intolerance*
Sudden change in diet*

Drugs/toxins

Acetazolamide
Adder bite
Allopurinol
Alpha-2 agonists
Aminophylline
Amphotericin B
Apomorphine
Aspirin
Atipamezole
Atropine
Batteries
Benzalkonium chloride
Bethanechol
Blue-green algae
Borax
Bromocriptine
Calcium edetate
Carbimazole
Carboplatin
Cardiac glycosides
Cephalexin
Chlorambucil
Chloramphenicol
Chlorphenamine
Clomipramine
Colchicine
Cotoneaster
Cyclophosphamide
Cyclosporin
Cytarabine
Daffodil
Dichlorophen
Diclofenac sodium
Dinoprost tromethamine
Dopamine
Doxorubicin
Doxycycline
Dieffenbachia
Ethylene glycol

Erythromycin
Glipizide
Glucocorticoids
Glyphosphate
Honeysuckle
Horse chestnut
Hydralazine
Ibuprofen
Indomethacin
Ipecacuanha
Iron/iron salts
Ivermectin
Ketoconazole
Laburnum
Lead
Levamisole
Lignocaine
Loperamide
Medetomidine
Melphalan
Metaldehyde
Methimazole
Metronidazole
Mexiletine
Misoprostol
Mistletoe
Mitotane
Naproxen
Nicotinamide
Nitroscanate
NPK fertilisers
NSAIDs
Paracetamol
Paraquat
Penicillamine
Pentoxifylline
Petroleum distillates
Phenoxy acid herbicides
Phenytoin
Pimobendan

Piperazine
Plastic explosives
Poinsettia
Potassium bromide
Procainamide
Propantheline bromide
Pyracantha
Pyrethrin/pyrethroids
Pyridostigmine
Rhododendron
Rowan
Salt
Selective serotonin reuptake inhibitors
Sildenafil
Sotalol
Strychnine
Sulphasalazine
Terfenadine
Tetracycline
Theobromine
Theophylline
Tricyclic antidepressants
Trimethoprim/sulphonamide
Ursodeoxycholic acid
Vitamin D rodenticides
Xylazine
Yew
Zinc

Endocrine disease, e.g.

Diabetic ketoacidosis*
Hypoadrenocorticism (D)

Gastrointestinal disease

Colitis*
Constipation/obstipation* *q.v.*
Foreign body*
Gastric dilatation/volvulus*
Gastric or duodenal ulceration*
Gastritis/enteritis*

Haemorrhagic gastroenteritis*
Infection, e.g.
- Bacterial*
- Parasites*
- Viral*

Inflammatory bowel disease*
Intestinal volvulus
Intussusception
Neoplasia*

Metabolic/systemic disease

Hypercalcaemia/hypocalcaemia *q.v.*
Hyperkalaemia/hypokalaemia* *q.v.*
Hyperthermia* *q.v.*
Liver disease* *q.v.*
Pancreatitis*
Peritonitis*
Prostatitis*
Pyometra* (D)
Renal disease* *q.v.*
Septicaemia*
Urinary obstruction*
Vestibular disease*

Miscellaneous conditions

Central nervous system disease
Diaphragmatic hernia
Motion sickness*
Psychogenic

CHRONIC VOMITING
Endocrine disease, e.g.

Diabetes mellitus*
Hyperthyroidism* (C)
Hypoadrenocorticism (D)

Gastrointestinal disease

Bacterial overgrowth
Colitis*

Constipation/obstipation* *q.v.*
Enterogastric reflux
Gastric motility disorders*
Gastric or duodenal ulceration*
Gastritis/enteritis*
Infection, e.g.
- Bacterial
- Fungal
- Parasites*
- Viral

Inflammatory bowel disease
- Eosinophilic
- Lymphocytic
- Lymphoplasmacytic
- Mixed

Irritable bowel syndrome
Neoplasia*
- Intestinal, e.g. lymphoma and adenocarcinoma
- Gastrinoma
- Mast cell tumour

Obstruction, e.g.
- Foreign body*
- Inflammatory bowel disease (gastritis or enteritis)
- Intussusception*
- Neoplasia*
- Pyloric stenosis
- Ulceration

Metabolic/systemic disease

Heartworm disease
Hypercalcaemia/hypocalcaemia *q.v.*
Hyperkalaemia/hypokalaemia *q.v.*
Liver disease* *q.v.*
Pancreatitis*
Prostatitis
Pyometra* (D)
Renal disease* *q.v.*
Septicaemia

Miscellaneous conditions

Abdominal neoplasia
Diaphragmatic hernia
Sialadenitis
Hydrocephalus
Brain tumour

1.2.6   Diarrhoea

SMALL INTESTINAL DIARRHOEA

Diet

Dietary intolerance, e.g.
Food hypersensitivity*
Food intolerance
Gluten-sensitive enteropathy

Overfeeding

Sudden change in diet

Drugs/toxins (see Large intestinal diarrhoea)

Extra-gastrointestinal disease

Exocrine pancreatic insufficiency*
Hepatic disease* *q.v.*
Hyperthyroidism* (C)
Hypoadrenocorticism (D)
IgA deficiency
Nephrotic syndrome
Pancreatic duct obstruction
Pancreatitis*
Renal disease* *q.v.*
Right-sided congestive heart failure*
Systemic lupus erythematosus
Uraemia

Idiopathic disease

Lymphangiectasia

Infection

Bacterial*, e.g.
  Campylobacter spp.
  Clostridium spp.
  E. coli
  Salmonella spp.
  Staphylococcus spp.
  Small intestinal bacterial overgrowth/antibiotic-responsive
  diarrhoea

Fungal

Helminths*
  Hookworm
  Roundworm
  Tapeworm
  Whipworm

Protozoal*, e.g.
  Cryptosporidiosis
  • *Giardia* spp.

Rickettsial

Viral*, e.g.
  Coronavirus
  Feline leukaemia virus (C)
  Parvovirus

Inflammatory/immune-mediated disease
  Basenji enteropathy (D)
  Duodenal ulceration
  Haemorrhagic gastroenteritis*
  Inflammatory bowel disease*
    • Eosinophilic
    • Granulomatous
    • Lymphoplasmacytic
  Protein-losing enteropathy and nephropathy
  of the soft-coated wheaten terrier (D)

Motility disorders, e.g.

Dysautonomia
Enteritis
Functional obstruction (ileus)
Hypoalbuminaemia
Hypokalaemia

Neoplasia*, e.g.

Adenocarcinoma
Carcinoid tumours
Leiomyoma
Lymphoma
Mast cell tumours
Sarcoma

Partial obstruction

Foreign body
Intussusception
Neoplasia
Stricture

LARGE INTESTINAL DIARRHOEA

Diet*

Dietary hypersensitivity
Dietary indiscretion

Drugs/toxins

Acetazolamide
Adder bite
Allopurinol
Aminophylline
Amoxicillin
Amphotericin B
Ampicillin
Atenolol
Benzalkonium chloride
Bethanechol
Blue-green algae
Borax

Calcium edetate
Carbamate insecticides
Cardiac glycosides
Cephalexin
Chloramphenicol
Chlorphenamine
Colchicine
Cotoneaster
Cyclophosphamide
Cyclosporin
Cytarabine
Daffodil
Diazoxide
Diclofenac sodium
Dieffenbachia
Doxycycline
Glyphosphate
Honeysuckle
Horse chestnut
Ibuprofen
Indomethacin
Iron/iron salts
Laburnum
Lactulose
Levamisole
Lithium
Loperamide
Mebendazole
Metaldehyde
Methiocarb
Misoprostol
Mistletoe
Mitotane
Naproxen
Nicotinamide
NPK fertilisers
NSAIDs
Organophosphates
Oxytetracycline
Pamidronate

Pancreatic enzyme supplementation
Paracetamol
Paraquat
Pentoxifylline
Petroleum distillates
Phenoxy acid herbicides
Piperazine
Poinsettia
Procainamide
Pyracantha
Pyrethrin/pyrethroids
Pyridostigmine
Quinidine
Rhododendron
Rowan
Salt
Selective serotonin reuptake inhibitors
Sotalol
Theobromine
Theophylline
Vitamin D rodenticides
Yew
Zinc sulphate

Extra-intestinal conditions

Metastatic neoplasia
Neurological disease leading to ulcerative colitis
Pancreatitis
Toxaemia
Uraemia

Idiopathic conditions

Fibre-responsive large-bowel diarrhoea
Irritable bowel syndrome

Infection

Bacterial*, e.g.
   Campylobacter spp.
   Clostridium difficile

Clostridium perfringens
E. coli
Salmonella spp.
Yersinia enterocolitica

Fungal, e.g.
Histoplasmosis
Protothecosis

Parasitic*, e.g.
Amoebiasis
Ancylostoma spp.
Balantidium coli
Cryptosporidiosis
Giardia spp.
Heterobilharzia americana
Roundworm
Tapeworm
Tritrichomonas foetus (C)
Uncinaria spp.
Whipworm

Protozoal, e.g.
Toxoplasmosis

Viral*
Coronavirus
Feline immunodeficiency virus (C)
Feline infectious peritonitis (C)
Feline leukaemia virus (C)
Parvovirus

Inflammatory/Immune-mediated disease

Histiocytic ulcerative colitis or granulomatous
colitis of boxers (and other breeds) (D)
Inflammatory bowel disease*

Neoplasia*

Benign, e.g.
Adenomatous polyps
Leiomyoma

Malignant, e.g.
    Adenocarcinoma
    Lymphoma

Obstruction
    Caecal inversion
    Foreign body*
    Intussusception*
    Neoplasia
    Stricture

Miscellaneous
    Secondary to chronic small intestinal disease
    Stress
Note: Perirectal diseases, e.g. anal sac disease, anal furunculosis, perineal hernia, rectal prolapse and perianal adenoma, may cause signs mimicking large-bowel disease (tenesmus, haematochezia, mucoid stool).

1.2.7   Melaena

Extra-gastrointestinal disease
    Hypoadrenocorticism (D)
    Liver disease* *q.v.*
    Mastocytosis
    Pancreatitis*
    Septicaemia*
    Shock* *q.v.*
    Systemic hypertension* *q.v.*
    Uraemia* *q.v.*
    Vasculitis, e.g.
        • Rocky Mountain spotted fever

Coagulopathy q.v., e.g.
    Anticoagulant toxicity* *q.v.*
    Congenital clotting factor deficiency *q.v.*
    Disseminated intravascular coagulation
    Thrombocytopenia *q.v.*
    Thrombocytopathia
    von Willebrand's disease (D)

Gastrointestinal disease
Enteritis*
Gastritis*
Oesophagitis
Parasites*

Gastrointestinal ulceration *
Gastrinoma
Helicobacter infection
Inflammatory gastroenteric disease*
Neurological disease
Post foreign body*
Stress
Uraemia* *q.v.*
Drugs, e.g.
* Glucocorticoids*
* NSAIDs*

Ischaemia, e.g.
Mesenteric avulsion
Mesenteric thrombosis/infarction
Mesenteric volvulus
Post gastric dilatation/volvulus* (D)

Neoplasia, e.g.*
Adenocarcinoma
Leiomyoma
Leiomyosarcoma
Lymphoma

Ingestion of blood

Nasal disease (see also Epistaxis), e.g.
Coagulopathy* *q.v.*
Neoplasia*
Trauma*

Oropharyngeal haemorrhage
Coagulopathy* *q.v.*
Neoplasia*
Trauma*

Respiratory disease (see also Haemoptysis), e.g.
    Coagulopathy* *q.v.*
    Exercise-induced pulmonary haemorrhage
    Parasites, e.g. *Angiostrongylus vasorum*
    Neoplasia*
    Ruptured aneurysm
    Trauma*

1.2.8   Haematemesis

Extra-gastrointestinal disease
    Hypoadrenocorticism (D)
    Liver disease* *q.v.*
    Mastocytosis
    Pancreatic disease
    Septicaemia*
    Shock*
    Systemic hypertension* *q.v.*
    Uraemia* *q.v.*

Coagulopathies q.v., e.g.
    Anticoagulant toxicity*
    Congenital clotting factor deficiency
    Disseminated intravascular coagulation
    Thrombocytopenia
    Thrombocytopathia
    von Willebrand's disease(D)

Toxins, e.g.
    Calcipotriol
    Paraquat

Vasculitis, e.g.
    Rocky Mountain spotted fever

Gastrointestinal disease
    Gastritis*
    Haemorrhagic gastroenteritis
    Oesophagitis

Gastrointestinal ulceration*
   Drugs, e.g.
      • NSAIDs
      • Glucocorticoids*
   Gastrinoma
   Helicobacter infection*
   Inflammatory gastroenteric disease*
   Neurological disease
   Post foreign body*
   Stress
   Systemic mastocytosis
   Uraemia*

Ischaemia, e.g.
   Post gastric dilatation/volvulus* (D)

Neoplasia*, e.g.
      • Adenocarcinoma
      • Lymphoma

Ingestion of blood

Nasal disease (see also Epistaxis), e.g.
   Coagulopathy* *q.v.*
   Infection, e.g. fungal
   Neoplasia*
   Trauma*

Oropharyngeal haemorrhage
   Coagulopathy* *q.v.*
   Neoplasia*
   Trauma*

Respiratory disease (see also Haemoptysis), e.g.
   Coagulopathy* *q.v.*
   Exercise-induced pulmonary haemorrhage
   Parasites
   Neoplasia*
   Ruptured aneurysm
   Trauma*

1.2.9 Haematochezia

Drugs
Glucocorticoids

Extra-gastrointestinal disease
Neurological disease leading to ulcerative colitis

Coagulopathies q.v., e.g.
Anticoagulant toxicity*
Congenital clotting factor deficiency *q.v.*
Disseminated intravascular coagulation
Thrombocytopenia *q.v.*
von Willebrand's disease (D)

Perirectal disease, e.g.
Anal furunculosis*
Anal sac disease*
Perianal adenoma*
Perineal hernia*
Rectal prolapse*

Gastrointestinal disease

Algal, e.g.
Prototheocosis

Bacterial, e.g.*
Campylobacter spp.
Clostridium spp.
E. coli
Salmonella spp.

Dietary
Dietary hypersensitivity
Dietary indiscretion

Fungal, e.g.
Histoplasmosis

Idiopathic conditions

Fibre-responsive large-bowel diarrhoea
Caecal disease, e.g.
- Typhlitis
- Inversion

Haemorrhagic gastroenteritis
Irritable bowel syndrome

Inflammatory/immune-mediated disease

Histiocytic ulcerative colitis or granulomatous colitis
of boxers (and other breeds) (D)
Inflammatory bowel disease*

Neoplasia

- *Benign, e.g.*
  - Adenomatous polyps
  - Leiomyoma
- *Malignant, e.g.*
  - Adenocarcinoma
  - Lymphoma

Obstructive disease

Foreign body*
Intussusception*

Parasitic*, e.g.

Amoebiasis
Ancylostoma spp.
Balantidium coli
Cryptosporidiosis
Giardia spp.
Heterobilharzia americana
Roundworm
Tapeworm
- Toxoplasmosis

Tritrichomonas foetus (C)
Uncinaria spp.
Whipworm

Viral*
Coronavirus
Feline immunodeficiency virus (C)
Feline infectious peritonitis (C)
Feline leukaemia virus (C)
Parvovirus

1.2.10   Constipation/obstipation

Behavioural factors*, e.g.
Change of daily routine
Dirty litter box
Hospitalisation
Inadequate water intake
Inadequate exercise
Novel litter substrate

Congenital conditions
Atresia ani
Atresia coli

Diet
Ingestion of hair, bones and foreign material
Low-fibre diets

Drugs/toxins
Aluminium antacids
Butylscopolamine (hyoscine)
Diphenoxylate
Diuretics
Loperamide
Opioids
Propantheline bromide
Sucralfate
Verapamil
Vincristine

Idiopathic conditions
Idiopathic megacolon*

Neuromuscular disease

Feline dysautonomia (C) (also reported rarely in dogs)
Lumbosacral disease*
Pelvic nerve disease, e.g.
- Traumatic*

Obstructive disease

Intraluminal/intramural

Diverticulum
Foreign body*
Neoplasia*, e.g.
- Adenoma
- Leiomyoma
- Leiomyosarcoma
- Lymphoma

Stricture

Extraluminal

Granuloma
Neoplasia*
Pelvic fracture*
Perineal hernia*
Prostatic disease (D)
- Abscess
- Benign prostatic hypertrophy*
- Neoplasia
- Prostatitis*

Sublumbar lymph node disease

Painful conditions

Anal furunculosis*
Anal or rectal inflammation*
Anal or rectal mass*
Anal or rectal stricture
Anal sac disease*, e.g.
- Abscess
- Anal sacculitis

Orthopaedic disease causing pain and failure to posture
Pelvic trauma (soft tissue or bony)*

Perianal fistula
Proctitis
Spinal cord disease*

Prolonged colonic distension, e.g.
Narrowing of the pelvic canal post fracture*

Systemic disease
Dehydration*
Hypercalcaemia *q.v.*
Hypokalaemia* *q.v.*
Hypothyroidism* (D)
Hyperparathyroidism

1.2.11   Faecal tenesmus/dyschezia

Anal sac disease, e.g.
Abscess/cellulitis
Anal sacculitis*
Impaction
Neoplasia
Stricture

Caudal abdominal mass*

Colorectal disease, e.g.
Colitis *q.v.*
Congenital disease
Foreign body
Large intestinal neoplasia
Megacolon
Polyp
Stricture

Constipation/obstipation *q.v.*

Diet
Excess bone
Excess fibre

Perianal disease, e.g.
Anal furunculosis/perianal fistulas* (D)
Perianal adenoma*
Perineal hernia*
Rectal prolapse*

Pelvic narrowing

Prostatic disease (D)
Abscess
Benign prostatic hypertrophy*
Neoplasia
Paraprostatic cyst
Prostatitis*

Trauma, e.g.
Pelvic fracture*

Urogenital disease*, e.g.
Lower urinary tract disease
Urethral obstruction

1.2.12 Faecal incontinence

Anal sphincter incompetence
Myopathy
Neoplasia*
Trauma*

Iatrogenic disease, e.g.
Damage to anal sphincter during anal sacculectomy

Neurological, e.g.
Cauda equina syndrome
Degenerative myelopathy/CDRM* (D)
Distemper encephalomyelitis
Dysautonomia
Lumbosacral stenosis
Myelodysplasia/spinal dysraphism

Peripheral neuropathy
Polyneuropathy
Sacrocaudal dysgenesis
Spinal arachnoid cysts
Spinal trauma

Perianal disease, e.g.
Perianal fistula*
Neoplasia

Reservoir incontinence
Behavioural
CNS disease *q.v.*
Colitis*
Constipation
Diet*
Neoplasia*
Perineal hernia

1.2.13   Flatulence/borborygmus

Aerophagia*
Competitive/aggressive eating
Nervous animal

Diet
High-fibre diets
Milk products/lactase deficiency
Spoiled food

Drugs/toxins, e.g.
Lactulose
Metaldehyde

Maldigestion, e.g.
Exocrine pancreatic insufficiency

Malabsorption, e.g.
Inflammatory bowel disease

1.3 Cardiorespiratory historical signs

1.3.1 Coughing

Drugs/toxins/irritants
Benzalkonium chloride ingestion
Chemical fume inhalation
Potassium bromide (C)
Smoke inhalation

Infection

Bacterial, e.g.
Bordetellosis*
  • Mycoplasma

Fungal, e.g.
Coccidioidomycosis

Viral, e.g.
Canine distemper*

Parasitic
Aelurostrongylus abstrusus (C)
Angiostrongylus vasorum (D)
Dirofilaria immitis
Oslerus osleri (D)
Paragonimiasis

Inflammatory/immune-mediated disease
Asthma* (C)
Chronic bronchitis*

Miscellaneous conditions
Aspiration pneumonia
Idiopathic pulmonary fibrosis
Inhaled foreign body
Laryngeal paralysis

Left atrial enlargement*
Lung lobe torsion
Primary ciliary dyskinesia

Neoplasia
Adenocarcinoma
Alveolar carcinoma
Bronchial gland carcinoma
Metastatic disease
Squamous cell carcinoma

Pulmonary haemorrhage
Coagulopathy *q.v.*
Exercise induced
Neoplasia*
Traumatic
   * *Angiostrongylus vasorum (D)*

Pulmonary oedema (D)
Airway obstruction
Cardiogenic*
Electrocution
Hypoglycaemia
Hypoproteinaemia *q.v.*
Iatrogenic
Ketamine
Neurological
   * Cranial trauma
   * Seizures
Obstruction of lymphatic drainage
Primary alveolar–capillary membrane injury
Re-expansion
Strangulation

1.3.2   Dyspnoea/tachypnoea

See Section 2.3.1.

1.3.3 Sneezing and nasal discharge

Anatomical deformities
Acquired nasopharyngeal stenosis
Cleft palate
Oronasal fistula

Congenital disease
Ciliary dyskinesia

Dental disease
Tooth root abscess*

Infection

Bacterial
Bordetella bronchiseptica *
Chlamydophila spp.*
Coliforms
Mycoplasma spp.
Pasteurella spp.
Staphylococcus spp.
Streptococcus spp.

Fungal
Aspergillosis
Cryptococcosis
Exophiala jeanselmei
Penicillium spp.
Phaeohyphomycosis
Rhinosporidium seeberi

Parasitic
Cuterebra spp.
Eucoleus böehmi
Linguatula serrata
Pneumonyssoides caninum

Viral
Canine distemper virus* (D)
Canine infectious tracheobronchitis* (D)

Feline calicivirus* (C)
Feline herpesvirus* (C)
Feline immunodeficiency virus* (C)
Feline leukaemia virus* (C)
Feline poxvirus
Feline reovirus (C)

Inflammatory disease
Allergic rhinitis*
Granulomatous rhinitis
Lymphoplasmacytic rhinitis*
Nasopharyngeal polyp* (C)

Neoplasia
Adenocarcinoma*
Chondrosarcoma
Fibrosarcoma
Haemangiosarcoma
Lymphoma*
Mast cell tumour
Melanoma
Neuroblastoma
Osteosarcoma
Squamous cell carcinoma*
Transmissible venereal tumour
Undifferentiated carcinomas*

Physical
Foreign body*
Irritant gases
Trauma

Systemic disease (see also Epistaxis)
Coagulopathy *q.v.*
Hypertension *q.v.*
Hyperviscosity syndrome
Vasculitis
- Ehrlichiosis
- Rocky Mountain spotted fever

1.3.4   Epistaxis

Coagulopathies q.v.
Angiostrongylus vasorum infection
Coagulation factor deficiency *q.v.*
Platelet disease
- Thrombocytopathia *q.v.*
- Thrombocytopenia *q.v.*

Miscellaneous conditions
Hypertension *q.v.*
Hyperviscosity syndrome e.g.
- Hyperlipidaemia,
- Polycythaemia
Increased capillary fragility
Thromboembolism

Nasal disease

Dental disease
Oronasal fistula
Tooth root abscess*

Infection
Bacterial
- *Mycoplasma* spp.*
- *Pasteurella* spp.*
Fungal
- Aspergillosis
- *Cryptococcus* spp.
- *Exophiala jeanselmei*
- *Penicillium* spp.
- Phaeohyphomycosis
- *Rhinosporidium seeberi*
Parasitic
- *Cuterebra*
- *Eucoleus böehmi*
- *Linguatula serrata*
- *Pneumonyssoides caninum*

Viral
- Canine distemper virus* (D)
- Canine infectious tracheobronchitis* (D)
- Feline calicivirus* (C)
- Feline herpesvirus* (C)
- Feline immunodeficiency virus* (C)
- Feline leukaemia virus* (C)

Inflammatory disease
Allergic rhinitis*
Lymphoplasmacytic rhinitis*

Neoplasia
Adenocarcinoma*
Chondrosarcoma
Fibrosarcoma
Haemangiosarcoma
Lymphoma*
Mast cell tumour
Melanoma
Osteosarcoma
Squamous cell carcinoma*
Transmissible venereal tumour
Undifferentiated carcinomas*

Physical
Trauma*

1.3.5 Haemoptysis

Cardiovascular disease
Arteriovenous fistula
Bacterial endocarditis
Dirofilaria immitis (D)
Pulmonary oedema* *q.v.*

Iatrogenic
Diagnostic procedures, e.g.
- Bronchoalveolar lavage
- Bronchoscopy

- Lung aspirate
- Trans-tracheal wash

Endotracheal intubation*

Pulmonary disease

Pulmonary hypertension
Pulmonary thromboembolism

Infection

Bacterial
- Nocardiosis
- Pneumonia*
- Pulmonary abscessation

Fungal
- Blastomycosis
- Coccidioidomycosis
- Histoplasmosis

Parasitic
- *Aelurostrongylus abstrusus (C)*
- *Angiostrongylus (D)*
- *Capillaria aerophila*
- *Dirofilaria immitis (D)*
- *Paragonimus kellicotti*

Viral
- Infectious tracheobronchitis*

Inflammatory

Bronchiectasis
Bronchopneumonia
Chronic bronchitis* (D)
Pulmonary infiltrate with eosinophils

Neoplastic

Adenocarcinoma
Chondrosarcoma
Metastatic tumours*
Squamous cell carcinoma

Physical

Abscess
Bronchial gland carcinoma

Foreign body
Lung lobe torsion
Trauma, e.g.
  • Pulmonary contusions

Systemic disease
Coagulation factor deficiency *q.v.*
Thrombocytopathia *q.v.*
Thrombocytopenia *q.v.*

1.3.6   Exercise intolerance

Cardiovascular disease, (see Section 1.1.7) e.g.
Arrhythmias
Congestive heart failure*
Cyanotic heart disease *q.v.*
Myocardial dysfunction
Obstruction to ventricular outflow

Drugs, e.g.
Drugs causing hypotension

Metabolic/endocrine disease, e.g.
Anaemia*
Hyperthyroidism* (C)
Hypoadrenocorticism (D)
Hypoglycaemia *q.v.*
Hypokalaemic polymyopathy
Hypothyroidism* (D)
Malignant hyperthermia

Neuromuscular/musculoskeletal disease, e.g.
Botulism
Cervical myelopathy (D)
Coonhound paralysis
Ischaemic neuromyopathy* (C)
Intermittent claudication
Lumbosacral pain
Myasthenia gravis

Myopathies
- Congenital
- Hypokalaemic
- Toxic

Peripheral neuropathy *q.v.*
Polyarthritis
Polymyositis
Protozoal myositis
Tick paralysis

Respiratory disease q.v., e.g.

Idiopathic pulmonary fibrosis
Pleural effusion*
Pulmonary oedema*
Upper airway obstruction *q.v.*

1.4 Dermatological historical signs

1.4.1 Pruritus

Drugs/toxins

Methimazole
Paracetamol

Endocrine disorders

Calcinosis cutis*
Hyperthyroidism* (C)
Predisposing to pyoderma
- Hyperadrenocorticism
- Hypothyroidism* (D)

Environmental

Contact irritant dermatitis*
Sunburn/solar dermatitis*

Immune-mediated disease

Drug eruptions
Discoid lupus erythematosus
Systemic lupus erythematosus

Allergy/hypersensitivity
    Atopy*
    Contact allergy*
    Food hypersensitivity*
    Hormonal hypersensitivity (D)
    Parasite hypersensitivity*, e.g.
- Fleas
- Mosquitoes

Pemphigus complex
    Pemphigus erythematosus
    Pemphigus foliaceus
    Pemphigus vegetans
    Pemphigus vulgaris
    Bullous pemphigoid

Infection

Bacterial
    Deep pyoderma*
    Surface pyoderma/acute moist dermatitis (wet eczema*)
    Superficial bacterial folliculitis*

Fungal
    Candidiasis
    Dermatophytosis*
    Malassezia dermatitis*
    Pythiosis

Parasitic
    Cheyletiellosis
    Demodicosis*
    Dermanyssus gallinae
    Dirofilariasis
    Dracunculiasis
    Fleas*
    Hookworm dermatitis
    Lynxacarus radovskyi (C)
    Notoedres cati (C)
    Otobius megnini (D)
    Otodectes cynotis
    Pediculosis
    Pelodera dermatitis

Pneumonyssoides caninum (D)
Sarcoptic mange* (D)
Schistosomiasis
Trombiculiasis*

Keratinisation disorders
Acne*
Idiopathic facial dermatitis
Primary seborrhoea
Vitamin A-responsive dermatosis

Miscellaneous
Feline hypereosinophilic syndrome (C)
Idiopathic sterile granulomatous dermatitis
Sterile eosinophilic pustulosis
Subcorneal pustular dermatosis
Urticaria pigmentosa
Waterline disease of black Labradors (D)
Zinc-responsive dermatosis

Neoplasia
Cutaneous T cell lymphoma
Mast cell tumour*
Mycosis fungoides
Other neoplasia with secondary pyoderma
Paraneoplastic pruritus

Neurological, e.g.
Syringohydromyelia

1.5   Neurological historical signs

1.5.1   Seizures

INTRACRANIAL
Congenital
Ceroid lipofuscinosis
Chiari-like malformation
Cortical dysplasia

Hydrocephalus
Intracranial arachnoid cysts
Lissencephaly
Lysosomal storage diseases
Organic acidurias, e.g.
- L-2-hydroxyglutaricaciduria

Idiopathic*
Infectious

Bacterial, e.g.
Nocardiosis
Pasteurella spp.
Staphylococcus spp.

Fungal
Aspergillosis
Blastomycosis
Coccidioidomycosis
Cryptococcosis
Histoplasmosis
Mucormycosis

Parasitic
Aberrant migration of *Cuterebra* spp.
Dirofilariasis

Protozoal, e.g.
Neosporosis (D)
Toxoplasmosis

Rickettsial encephalitis
Ehrlichiosis/anaplasmosis
Rocky Mountain spotted fever

Viral
Canine distemper* (D)
Canine herpesvirus (D)
Eastern equine encephalitis
Feline immunodeficiency virus* (C)

Feline infectious peritonitis* (C)
Feline leukaemia virus* (C)
Pseudorabies
Rabies

Inflammatory/immune-mediated disease

Breed-specific necrotising
meningoencephalitis
Distemper vaccine associated (D)
Eosinophilic meningoencephalitis
Granulomatous meningoencephalomyelitis* (D)
Steroid-responsive meningoencephalitis

Neoplasia

Local extension

Middle-ear tumour
Nasal/paranasal sinus tumour
Pituitary tumour
Skull tumour

Metastatic, e.g.

Haemangiosarcoma
Lymphoma
Malignant melanoma
Mammary carcinoma
Prostatic carcinoma
Pulmonary carcinoma
Teratoma

Primary intracranial

Astrocytoma
Choroid plexus tumours
Ependymoma
Ganglioblastoma
Glioma
Medulloblastoma
Meningioma
Neuroblastoma
Oligodendroglioma

Physical
Trauma

Vascular

Haemorrhage, e.g.
Angiostrongylus vasorum
Coagulopathy *q.v.*
Feline ischaemic encephalopathy (C)
Hypertension *q.v.*
Trauma

Infarction, e.g.
Thromboembolism

EXTRACRANIAL

Drugs/toxins
Alphachloralose
Arsenic
Baclofen
Blue-green algae
Borax
Cannabis
Carbamate
Doxapram
Ethylene glycol
Glyphosphate
Honeysuckle
Hymenoptera stings
Ibuprofen
Iodine-containing myelographic contrast media
Laburnum
Lead
Lignocaine
Metaldehyde
Metronidazole
Mexiletine
Mistletoe
Organophosphates
Paracetamol

Petroleum distillates
Phenoxy acid herbicides
Piperazine
Plastic explosives
Pyrethrin/pyrethroids/permethrin
Risperidone
Salt
Selective serotonin reuptake inhibitors
Strychnine
Terfenadine
Theobromine
Theophylline
Tricyclic antidepressants
Vitamin D rodenticides
Yew

Metabolic
Electrolyte imbalances*, e.g.
- Hypernatraemia *q.v.*
- Hypocalcaemia *q.v.*
- Hyponatraemia *q.v.*

Hepatic encephalopathy* *q.v.*
- Hypoglycaemia *q.v.*
- Renal disease* *q.v.*

Nutritional
Thiamine deficiency

1.5.2   Trembling/shivering

Drugs/toxins
5-Fluorouracil
Baclofen
Benzodiazepines
Blue-green algae
Bromethalin
Caffeine
Carbamate

Guarana
Hexachlorophene
Horse chestnut
Ivermectin
Macadamia nuts
Metaldehyde
Mexiletine
Mycotoxins
Risperidone
Organochlorines
Organophosphates
Petroleum distillates
Plastic explosives
Piperazine
Pyrethrin/pyrethroids/permethrin
Rhododendron
Salbutamol
Salt
Strychnine
Terbutaline
Theobromine
Theophylline
Tricyclic antidepressants
Yew
Zinc phosphate

Metabolic

Hepatic encephalopathy *q.v.**
Hyperadrenocorticism/hypoadrenocorticism (D)
Hyperkalaemia *q.v.*
Hypocalcaemia *q.v.*
Hypoglycaemia *q.v.*
Primary hyperparathyroidism
Uraemia *q.v.**

Neurological

Abiotrophies
Cerebellar disease *q.v.*
Central nervous system inflammatory disease
Cerebrospinal hypomyelinogenesis and dysmyelinogenesis
Corticosteroid responsive tremor syndrome ('white dog shaker disease')

Idiopathic head nod of Dobermanns and bulldogs
Lumbosacral disease, e.g.
- Disc herniation
- Discospondylitis
- Neoplasia
- Stenosis

Lysosomal storage disease
Neuroaxonal dystrophy (D)
Nerve root compression
Niemann–Pick disease (C)
Peripheral neuropathies *q.v.*
Primary orthostatic tremor
Senility
Spongiform encephalopathy

Physiological

Ballistocardiographic*
Fatigue/weakness*
Fear*
Reduced environmental temperature*

1.5.3 Ataxia

FOREBRAIN

Congenital

Dandy–Walker syndrome
Hydrocephalus
Intra-arachnoid cyst

Degenerative

Leukodystrophy
Lysosomal storage disease
Mitochondrial encephalopathy
Multi-system neuronal degeneration
Spongy degeneration

Immune-mediated disease/infection

Encephalitis *q.v.*
Feline spongiform encephalopathy

Metabolic

Electrolyte/acid–base disorders *q.v.**
Hepatic encephalopathy *q.v.**
Hypoglycaemia *q.v.*
Uraemic encephalopathy *q.v.**

Neoplasia

Choroid plexus tumours
Dermoid cyst
Ependymoma
Epidermoid cyst
Glioma
Lymphoma
Medulloblastoma
Meningioma
Metastatic tumour

Vascular

Cerebrovascular accident

BRAINSTEM/CENTRAL VESTIBULAR DISORDERS

Congenital

Chiari-like malformation
Hydrocephalus
Intra-arachnoid cysts

Degenerative

Lysosomal storage disorders

Drugs

Metronidazole

Immune mediated/infectious

Feline spongiform encephalopathy (C)
Meningoencephalitis *q.v.*

Metabolic

Electrolyte abnormalities* *q.v.*
Hepatic encephalopathy* *q.v.*
Uraemic encephalopathy* *q.v.*

Neoplastic
Choroid plexus tumours
Dermoid cyst
Epidermoid cyst
Glioma
Lymphoma
Medulloblastoma
Meningioma
Metastatic tumour

Nutritional
Thiamine deficiency

Trauma

Vascular
Cerebrovascular accident

CEREBELLUM (generally ataxia without conscious proprioceptive deficits)

Congenital
Feline cerebellar hypoplasia (C)

Degenerative
Cerebellar cortical degeneration
Gangliosidosis
Hereditary ataxia of Jack Russell and smooth-coated
fox terriers (D)
Leukoencephalomalacia (D)
Neuroaxonal dystrophy (D)
Neuronal vacuolation and spinocerebellar degeneration (D)
Storage diseases

Drugs/toxins
Heavy metals
Organophosphates

Immune mediated/infectious *q.v.*
In utero infection with feline parvovirus (C)

Metabolic
Thiamine deficiency

Neoplastic
Choroid plexus tumours
Dermoid cyst
Epidermoid cyst
Glioma
Lymphoma
Medulloblastoma
Meningioma
Metastatic tumour

Vascular
Cerebrovascular accident *q.v.*

PERIPHERAL VESTIBULAR DISEASE

Congenital
Lymphocytic labyrinthitis
Non-inflammatory cochlear degeneration

Drugs/toxins
Aminoglycosides
Chlorhexidine
Topical iodophors

Idiopathic
Canine geriatric vestibular disease
Feline idiopathic vestibular disease

Immune mediated/infectious
Nasopharyngeal polyps*
Otitis media/interna*
- Primary secretory otitis media in the Cavalier King Charles Spaniel
- Secondary to otitis externa

Metabolic
Hypothyroidism* (D)

Neoplastic

Middle- or inner-ear tumours, e.g.
Adenocarcinoma
Chondrosarcoma
Fibrosarcoma
Lymphoma
Osteosarcoma
Squamous cell carcinoma

Traumatic

SPINE

Congenital

Atlanto-occipital dysplasia
Atlantoaxial subluxation
Cartilaginous exostoses
Dermoid sinus
Epidermoid cyst
Hereditary myelopathy
Meningocoeles
Sacral osteochondritis dissecans
Sacrocaudal dysgenesis
Spina bifida
Spinal arachnoid cyst
Spinal dysraphism
Syringohydromyelia (D)
Tethered cord syndrome
Vertebral malformations *q.v.*

Degenerative

Cervical fibrotic stenosis
Cervical spondylomyelopathy
Degenerative disc disease* (D)
Degenerative myelopathy*
Leukoencephalomalacia
Lumbosacral disease
Lysosomal storage disease
Neuroaxonal dystrophy
Neuronal vacuolation and spinocerebellar degeneration (D)

Other leukodystrophies
Synovial cysts

Idiopathic
Calcinosis circumscripta
Disseminated idiopathic skeletal hyperostosis

Immune mediated
Cauda equina neuritis
Granulomatous meningoencephalomyelitis*
Steroid-responsive meningitis–arteritis

Infectious
Discospondylitis
Foreign body
Meningomyelitis
Spinal epidural empyema

Neoplastic

Extradural
Chondrosarcoma
Fibrosarcoma
Haemangiosarcoma
Lipoma
Lymphoma
Malignant nerve sheath tumour
Meningioma
Metastatic disease
Myeloma
Osteosarcoma

Intradural extramedullary
Malignant nerve sheath tumour
Meningioma
Metastatic

Intramedullary
Astrocytoma
Ependymoma

Metastatic tumour
Oligodendroglioma

Nutritional
Hypervitaminosis A
Thiamine deficiency

Traumatic
Brachial plexus avulsion
Dural tear
Fracture*
Gunshot wound
Luxation*
Sacrocaudal injury
Traumatic disc injury*

Vascular
Fibrocartilaginous embolism*
Fat-graft necrosis
Myelomalacia
Spinal cord haematoma
Spinal cord haemorrhage
Vascular anomaly

PERIPHERAL NERVES (mono- or polyneuropathies)
Degenerative
Birman cat distal polyneuropathy (C)
Boxer dog progressive axonopathy (D)
Giant axonal neuropathy of German shepherds (D)
Globoid cell leukodystrophy
Golden retriever hypomyelinating polyneuropathy (D)
Hereditary/idiopathic polyneuropathy of Alaskan malamutes (D)
Hypertrophic neuropathy
Hypomyelinating polyneuropathy
Laryngeal paralysis–polyneuropathy complex
Lysosomal storage diseases
- Fucosidosis (D)
- Globoid cell leukodystrophy
- Glycogen storage disease type IV
- Niemann–Pick disease (C)

Mucopolysaccharidosis IIIA (D)
Sensory neuropathy (D)

Immune mediated/infectious

Chronic inflammatory demyelinating polyneuropathy
Feline leukaemia virus associated
Polyradiculoneuritis
Protozoal
Sensory ganglioradiculoneuritis

Neoplastic

Lymphoma
Malignant nerve sheath tumours
Myelomonocytic neoplasia
Paraneoplastic neuropathy

Traumatic

Bite wounds*
Iatrogenic
Missile injuries
Traction injuries

Vascular

Ischaemic neuromyopathy*
Neurogenic claudication

SYSTEMIC

Drugs/toxins

Alphachloralose
Baclofen
Benzodiazepines
Blue-green algae
Butorphanol
Cannabis
Carbamate
Codeine
Daffodil
Dichlorophen
Diclofenac

Ethylene glycol toxicity
Fentanyl and other sedatives and tranquillisers
Glyphosphate
Horse chestnut
Ivermectin
Loperamide
Metaldehyde
Methiocarb
Metronidazole
Naproxen
Nitroscanate (C)
Organophosphates
Paracetamol
Paraquat
Phenobarbitone
Phenoxy acid herbicides
Phenytoin
Piperazine
Plastic explosives
Potassium bromide
Primidone
Pyridoxine (Vitamin B6)
Selective serotonin reuptake inhibitors
Terfenadine
Thallium
Theobromine
Tricyclic antidepressants
Vincristine
Walker Hound mononeuropathy
Yew

Metabolic

Electrolyte/acid–base disorders*
Endocrine disease, e.g.
- Diabetes mellitus*
- Hypothyroidism* (D)

Hepatic encephalopathy*
Hyperadrenocorticoid neuropathy
Hyperchylomicronaemia
Insulinoma/hypoglycaemia

Nutritional
Vitamin B6 (pyridoxine) overdose

1.5.4 Paresis/paralysis

SPINAL DISEASE

Congenital
Atlantoaxial subluxation
Atlanto-occipital dysplasia
Cartilaginous exostoses
Dermoid sinus
Epidermoid cyst
Hereditary myelopathy
Meningocoeles
Osteochondromatosis
Sacrocaudal dysgenesis
Sacral osteochondritis dissecans
Spina bifida
Spinal arachnoid cyst
Spinal dysraphism
Syringohydromyelia (D)
Vertebral malformations *q.v.*

Degenerative
Afghan hound hereditary myelopathy (D)
Calcinosis circumscripta
Cervical spondylomyelopathy
Degenerative disc disease* (D)
Degenerative myelopathy* (D)
Labrador retriever axonopathy (D)
Lumbosacral disease
Lysosomal storage disease
Neuronal vacuolation and spinocerebellar degeneration (D)
Rottweiler leukoencephalomyelopathy (D)
Other leukodystrophies
Synovial cysts

Idiopathic
Calcinosis circumscripta
Disseminated idiopathic skeletal hyperostosis

Immune mediated

Cauda equina neuritis
Epidural granuloma
Granulomatous meningoencephalomyelitis*
Steroid-responsive meningitis–arteritis

Infectious

Discospondylitis
Infectious meningoencephalomyelitis
Spinal epidural empyema

Neoplastic

Extradural

Chondrosarcoma
Fibrosarcoma
Haemangiosarcoma
Lipoma
Lymphoma
Malignant nerve sheath tumour
Meningioma
Metastatic
Multiple myeloma
Osteosarcoma
Plasma cell tumour

Intradural extramedullary

Malignant nerve sheath tumour
Meningioma
Metastatic

Intramedullary

Astrocytoma
Ependymoma
Metastatic tumour
Oligodendroglioma

Nutritional

Hypervitaminosis A
Thiamine deficiency

Traumatic

Brachial plexus avulsion
Dural tear
Foreign body
Fracture*
Gunshot wound
Luxation*
Sacrocaudal injury
Traumatic disc injury*

Vascular

Fibrocartilaginous embolism*
Fat-graft necrosis
Ischaemic neuromyopathy*
Myelomalacia
Neurogenic claudication
Spinal cord haematoma
Spinal cord haemorrhage
Vascular anomaly

PERIPHERAL NERVES (mono- or polyneuropathies)

Degenerative

Adult-onset motor neurone disease
Birman cat distal polyneuropathy (C)
Boxer dog progressive axonopathy (D)
Distal denervating disease (D)
Giant axonal neuropathy of German shepherds (D)
Golden retriever hypomyelinating polyneuropathy (D)
Hereditary/idiopathic polyneuropathy of Alaskan malamutes (D)
Hypertrophic neuropathy
Idiopathic polyneuropathy
Laryngeal paralysis–polyneuropathy complex
Lysosomal storage diseases
- Fucosidosis (D)
- Globoid cell leukodystrophy
- Glycogen storage disease type IV
- Niemann–Pick disease (C)
Mucopolysaccharidosis IIIA (D)
Rottweiler distal sensorimotor polyneuropathy (D)

Sensory neuropathy of long-haired dachshunds (D)
Spinal muscular atrophy

Drugs/toxins

Baclofen
Blue-green algae
Cannabis
Daffodil
Horse chestnut
Ivermectin
Methiocarb
Organophosphate
Petroleum products
Phenoxy acid herbicides
Pyrethrin/pyrethroids
Salinomycin toxicity (C)
Thallium
Vincristine
Vitamin K antagonists
Walker hound mononeuropathy (D)

Immune mediated/infectious

Acute idiopathic polyradiculoneuritis (coonhound paralysis in the USA) (D)
Brachial plexus neuritis
Chronic inflammatory demyelinating polyneuropathy
Protozoal polyradiculoneuritis
Sensory ganglioradiculoneuritis

Metabolic

Diabetic neuropathy*
Hyperchylomicronaemia
Hypothyroid neuropathy*
Primary hyperoxaluria

Neoplastic

Insulinoma
Lymphoma
Malignant nerve sheath tumours
Myelomonocytic neoplasia
Paraneoplastic neuropathy, e.g. lymphoma

Traumatic
Bite wounds*
Iatrogenic
Missile injuries
Traction injuries

Vascular
Arterial thromboembolism
Ischaemic neuromyopathy*
Traumatic ischaemic neuromyopathy associated with bottom-hung pivot windows and garage doors

1.5.5 Coma/stupor

INTRACRANIAL DISEASE
(*Note:* Especially lesions of the midbrain through the medulla that impair the ascending reticular activating system)

Congenital
Hydrocephalus

Degenerative
Inherited neurodegenerative diseases
* Multi-system neuronal degeneration of cocker spaniels (D)
* Multi-systemic chromatolytic neuronal degeneration
* Spongiform degenerations

Inflammatory/infectious q.v.
Neoplastic

Local extension
Nasal tumour
Skull osteochondroma

Metastatic
Carcinoma
Haemangiosarcoma

Primary
> Choroid plexus papilloma
> Glioma
> Lymphoma
> Meningioma
> Pituitary tumour

Trauma
> Head trauma
> Intracranial haemorrhage
> Subdural haematoma

Vascular
> Cerebrovascular accident
> Feline ischaemic encephalopathy (C)
> Hypertension *q.v.*
> Intracranial haemorrhage

EXTRACRANIAL DISEASE

CNS perfusion disturbances
> Anaemia (severe/acute)* *q.v.*
> Cardiorespiratory disease*
> Haemoglobin-related toxicity
> Hyperviscosity
> Hypovolaemia (severe/acute)*

Drugs/toxins
> Alphachloralose
> Baclofen
> Barbiturates
> Benzodiazepines and other sedatives/anaesthetic agents
> Blue-green algae
> Borax
> Cannabis
> Carbamate insecticides
> Diclofenac sodium
> Ethylene glycol
> Ibuprofen
> Indomethacin

Iron
Ivermectin
Lead
Loperamide
Metaldehyde
Methiocarb
Metronidazole
Naproxen
Organophosphates
Paracetamol
Phenoxy acid herbicides
Salt
Tricyclic antidepressants
Vitamin K antagonists
Water
Xylitol
Yew

Metabolic

Electrolyte disturbances* *q.v.*
Hepatic encephalopathy*
Hypoglycaemia *q.v.*
Hypothyroid myxoedema coma
Uraemic encephalopathy *q.v.*

Nutritional

Thiamine deficiency

1.5.6　Altered behaviour: General changes

(E.g. disorientation, increased aggression, and loss of normal behaviour)

INTRACRANIAL DISEASE

Congenital

Hydrocephalus
Lissencephaly
Lysosomal storage diseases

Degenerative
Cognitive dysfunction

Drugs/toxins
Acepromazine
Benzodiazepines
Other sedatives/tranquillisers
Cannabis
Ibuprofen
Ivermectin
Petroleum distillates
Phenylpropanolamine
Risperidone
Salbutamol
Selective serotonin reuptake inhibitors
Selegiline
Terfenadine

Infectious

Bacterial

Fungal

Prion
Feline spongiform encephalopathy

Protozoal
Neosporosis
Toxoplasmosis

Viral
Canine distemper* (D)
Feline immunodeficiency virus* (C)
Feline infectious peritonitis* (C)
Feline leukaemia virus* (C)

Inflammatory/immune mediated
Granulomatous meningoencephalitis
Meningoencephalitis of unknown origin
Necrotising meningoencephalitis

Neoplastic, e.g.

Glioma
Lymphoma
Meningioma
Metastatic disease
Pituitary

Physical

Trauma

EXTRACRANIAL DISEASE

Metabolic

Hepatic encephalopathy *q.v.*
Hypocalcaemia *q.v.*
Hypoglycaemia *q.v.*
Renal disease *q.v.*
Thiamine deficiency

1.5.7 Altered behaviour: Specific behavioural problems

Aggression

Dominance*
Fear*
Hypocholesterolaemia
Petting*
Play*
Possessive*
Predatory*
Territorial*

Inappropriate urination and defecation

Cognitive dysfunction
Fear
Gastrointestinal disease *q.v.*
Hyperexcitability
Litter box related
  • Dirty litter

- New location of the litter box
- Unfamiliar litter

Separation anxiety
Territorial marking
Urinary tract disease (see Incontinence/inappropriate urination)

Stereotypy/compulsive behaviour
Boredom*
Frustration*
Genetic predisposition*
Physical triggers, e.g.
- Anal sac disease (tail chasing)*
- Dermatitis in over-grooming*

Neurological disease
- Brainstem lesions *q.v.*
- Forebrain disease *q.v.*
- Lumbosacral disease (tail chasing)
- Seizures* *q.v.*
- Sensory neuropathies (self-mutilation)
- Vestibular lesions (circling)* *q.v.*

Stress*

1.5.8 Deafness

Congenital conditions
Aplasia/hypoplasia of auditory receptors
Hydrocephalus

Degenerative disease
Presbycusis/age-related hearing loss*(D)
- Cochlear conductive defects
- Senile ossicle or receptor degeneration

Drugs/toxins

Antibiotics
Aminoglycosides
Amphotericin B
Ampicillin

Bacitracin
Chloramphenicol
Colistin
Erythromycin
Griseofulvin
Hygromycin B
Minocycline
Polymyxin B
Tetracyclines
Vancomycin

Antiseptics
Benzalkonium chloride
Benzethonium chloride
Cetrimide
Chlorhexidine
Ethanol
Iodine
Iodophors

Cancer chemotherapeutics
Actinomycin
Cisplatin
Cyclophosphamide
Vinblastine
Vincristine

Diuretics
Bumetanide
Ethacrynic acid
Frusemide

Metals/heavy metals
Arsenic
Gold salts
Lead
Mercury
Triethyl/trimethyl tin

Miscellaneous
Ceruminolytic agents
Danazol

Detergents
Digoxin
Dimethyl sulphoxide
Diphenylhydrazine
Insulin
Potassium bromide
Prednisolone
Propylene glycol
Quinidine
Salicylates

Idiopathic

Infection/inflammation

Otitis externa* *q.v.*
Otitis interna*
Otitis media*

Mechanical

Loud noise
Trauma

Neoplasia

Intracranial
Middle ear
Nasopharyngeal polyp*

1.5.9 Multifocal neurological disease

Congenital

Hydrocephalus
Syringohydromyelia

Degenerative

Mitochondrial encephalopathies
Organic acidurias
Storage diseases

Drugs/toxins

Alphachloralose

Baclofen
Benzodiazepines
Blue-green algae
Borax
Cannabis
Carbamate
Daffodil
Dichlorophen
Diclofenac sodium
Ethylene glycol
Glyphosphate
Horse chestnut
Ibuprofen
Ivermectin
Laburnum
Loperamide
Metaldehyde
Methiocarb
Naproxen
Organophosphates
Paracetamol
Petroleum products
Piperazine
Plastic explosives
Pyrethrin/pyrethroids
Rhododendron
Salbutamol
Salt
Selective serotonin reuptake inhibitors
Terfenadine
Theobromine
Tricyclic antidepressants
Vitamin D2/D3
Vitamin K antagonists
Yew

Idiopathic conditions

Dysautonomia

Immune-mediated disease

Granulomatous meningoencephalomyelitis

Necrotising encephalitis
Spinal cord vasculitis
Steroid-responsive meningitis–arteritis

Infectious

Bacterial
Bacterial encephalitis/meningitis
Tetanus

Fungal
Aspergillosis
Blastomycosis
Candidiasis
Coccidioidomycosis
Cryptococcosis

Parasitic
Cuterebra spp.
Toxocariasis

Protozoal
Neosporosis
Toxoplasmosis

Rickettsial
Ehrlichiosis/anaplasmosis
Prototothecosis
Rocky Mountain spotted fever

Viral
Canine distemper virus (D)*
Feline immunodeficiency virus* (C)
Feline infectious peritonitis* (C)
Feline leukaemia virus* (C)
Herpesvirus
Parainfluenza virus
Parvovirus*

Metabolic
Hepatic disease* *q.v.*

Hyperosmolarity
Hypoglycaemia *q.v.*
Hypothyroidism* (D)
Renal disease* *q.v.*

Neoplastic
Leukaemia
Lymphoma
Metastatic neoplasia

Nutritional
Thiamine deficiency

Vascular
Intracranial and/or spinal haemorrhage
* *Angiostrongylus vasorum*
* Coagulopathy
* Trauma
* Vascular anomaly
Hypertension *q.v.*
Thromboembolism

1.6 Ocular historical signs

1.6.1 Blindness/visual impairment

CENTRAL NERVOUS SYSTEM (CNS)
Brain disease

Congenital, e.g.
Hydrocephalus

Degenerative, e.g.
Neuronal ceroid lipofuscinosis
Lysosomal storage diseases

Drugs/toxins, e.g.
Ivermectin/moxidectin
Lead

Levamisole
Metaldehyde

Immune mediated/infectious, e.g.
Granulomatous meningoencephalomyelitis
Toxoplasmosis

Metabolic, e.g.
Hepatic encephalopathy *q.v.*

Neoplastic, e.g.
Lymphoma
Meningioma
Pituitary tumour

Trauma

Vascular, e.g.
Cerebrovascular accident

Optic nerve disease, e.g.
Optic nerve hypoplasia/aplasia
Optic neuritis
Space-occupying lesion compressing the optic nerve
Trauma

INTRAOCULAR/PERIOCULAR

Acquired
Anterior uveitis
Cataract* *q.v.*
Chorioretinitis
Chronic superficial keratitis/pannus*
Chronic uveitis*
Corneal lipid dystrophy/degeneration
Corneal oedema and endothelial dysfunction*
Endophthalmitis
Entropion
Generalised progressive retinal degeneration
Glaucoma*

Hypertensive ocular disease*
Hyphaema
Intraocular haemorrhage*
Keratoconjunctivitis sicca*
Nutritional retinal degeneration
  • Taurine deficiency
  • Vitamin A deficiency
  • Vitamin E deficiency
Phthisis bulbi, e.g.
  • Secondary to ocular trauma or chronic uveitis
Pigmentary keratitis
Retinal degeneration
Retinal detachment* *q.v.*
Retinal haemorrhage
Retinal pigment epithelial cell dystrophy
Sudden acquired retinal degeneration
Superficial keratitis
Symblepharon
Trauma*
Ulcerative keratitis and corneal scarring
Vitreal haemorrhage

Sequelae to chronic uveitis *
Corneal oedema
Cyclitic membranes
Exudative retinal detachment
Hyphaema
Intraocular adhesions
Lens luxation
Phthisis bulbi
Secondary cataracts
Secondary glaucoma
Secondary retinal degeneration*

Congenital
Ankyloblepharon
Anophthalmia
Anterior segment dysgenesis
Collie eye anomaly
Congenital vitreous opacification

Corneal dermoid
Entropion (severe)
Microphthalmia
Persistent hyperplastic primary vitreous
Persistent hyperplastic tunica vasculosa lentis
Persistent pupillary membranes
Posterior segment coloboma
Vitreo-retinal dysplasia

Lens disorders
Aphakia
Cataracts
Coloboma
Lenticonus/lentiglobus
Microphakia
Spherophakia

Retinal disorders
Congenital retinal dystrophy
Early-onset photoreceptor dystrophies
- Early retinal degeneration
- Photoreceptor dysplasia
- Rod–cone dysplasia
- Rod dysplasia
Hemeralopia
Lysosomal storage diseases
Primary retinal dysplasia
Secondary retinal dysplasia
- Idiopathic/inherited
- Intrauterine trauma
- Maternal infections
- Radiation
- Vitamin A deficiency during pregnancy

1.6.2 Epiphora/tear overflow

Impaired tear drainage
Dacryocystitis
Entropion

Imperforate/obstructed punctum
or canaliculus
Lacrimal canalicular aplasia
Small lacrimal lakes

Painful/irritating ocular conditions

Extraorbital conditions
Diseases of paranasal sinuses
Mechanical or olfactory stimulation
of the nasal mucosa

Eyelid conditions*
Blepharitis
Distichiasis/ectopic cilia
Entropion
Facial nerve paralysis
Lid laceration
Neoplasia
Trichiasis

Intraocular conditions
Acute uveitis
Anterior lens luxation (D)
Glaucoma
Trauma

Ocular surface conditions
Conjunctivitis*
Corneal ulceration*
Foreign body
Keratitis*

Third eyelid conditions*
Lymphoid hyperplasia
Neoplasia
Prolapsed nictitans gland
Scrolled third eyelid
Trauma

1.7 Musculoskeletal historical signs

1.7.1 Forelimb lameness

YOUNG ANIMALS

Any site
Infection*
Metaphyseal osteopathy
Panosteitis
Trauma*
- Bruising or strain of soft tissues*
- Laceration*
- Penetrating wound*

Shoulder
Brachial plexus avulsion
Fracture of the humerus*
Fracture of the scapula
Haemarthrosis
Joint capsule rupture
Luxation (congenital or acquired)
Medially displaced biceps tendon
Osteochondrosis* (D)
Septic arthritis*
Shoulder dysplasia*
Traumatic arthritis*

Elbow
Avulsion of the medial epicondyle
Collateral ligament rupture or avulsion
Degenerative joint disease*
Elbow incongruity
Fracture of the humerus*
Fracture of the radius*
Fracture of the ulna*
Growth plate disorders
Haemarthrosis

Luxation (congenital or acquired)
Osteochondrosis (D)*
- Fragmented medial coronoid process
- Osteochondritis dissecans of the medial condyle of the humerus
- Ununited anconeal process

Septic arthritis
Traumatic arthritis*

Carpus

Carpal hyperextension
Collateral ligament rupture or avulsion
Degenerative joint disease*
Dysostosis
Flexor tendon contracture
Fracture of the carpal bones*
Fracture of the metacarpal bones*
Fracture of the radius*
Fracture of the ulna*
Growth plate disorders
Luxation
Osteochondrosis
Septic arthritis
Shearing injury
Subluxation

Foot

Avulsion of the deep digital flexor tendon
Avulsion of the superficial digital flexor tendon
Claw disease *q.v.**
Degenerative joint disease*
Fracture of distal metacarpal bones*
Fracture of phalanges*
Injury to the integument, e.g.
- Bite wound
- Foreign body
- Laceration

Other pathology of the integument*
Luxation/subluxation
Septic arthritis
Sesamoid disease/fracture

ADULT ANIMALS

Any site
Infection*
Trauma*
- Bruising or strain of soft tissues
- Laceration
- Penetrating wound

Shoulder
Biceps tendon rupture
Bicipital tenosynovitis (D)
Degenerative joint disease*
Fracture of the humerus*
Fracture of the scapula*
Haemarthrosis
Infraspinatus contracture/other muscle contractures
Joint capsule rupture
Luxation (congenital or acquired)*
Medially displaced biceps tendon
Neoplasia*, e.g.
- Metastatic tumour
- Nerve root tumour
- Primary bone tumour
- Soft tissue tumour
- Synovial sarcoma
Osteochondrosis
Septic arthritis
Shoulder dysplasia
Traumatic arthritis*

Elbow
Collateral ligament rupture or avulsion
Degenerative joint disease*
Elbow incongruity
Fracture of the humerus*
Fracture of the radius*
Fracture of the ulna*
Haemarthrosis
Incomplete ossification of the humeral condyle

Luxation (congenital or acquired)
Medial spur
Neoplasia*
- Bone
- Metastatic
- Soft tissue
Osteochondrosis
Septic arthritis
Traumatic arthritis*

Carpus

Carpal hyperextension
Degenerative joint disease*
Fracture of the radius*
Fractures of the carpal bones*
Fractures of the metacarpal bones*
Haemarthrosis
Luxation or subluxation
Neoplasia*
- Bone
- Metastatic
- Soft tissue
Septic arthritis
Shearing injury
Traumatic arthritis*

Foot

Avulsion of the superficial or deep digital flexor tendon
Claw disease *q.v.*
Degenerative joint disease*
Fracture of the distal metacarpal bones*
Fracture of the phalanges*
Fracture of the sesamoid bones*
Haemarthrosis
Injury to the integument*, e.g.
- Bite wound
- Foreign body
- Laceration
Other pathology of the integument*
Luxation

Neoplasia
- Bone
- Metastatic
- Soft tissue

Septic arthritis
Sesamoid disease
Traumatic arthritis*

1.7.2 Hindlimb lameness

YOUNG ANIMALS

Any site
Infection
Metaphyseal osteopathy
Panosteitis
Trauma
- Bruising or strain of soft tissues
- Laceration
- Penetrating wound

Hip
Avascular necrosis of the femoral head (D)
Fracture of the acetabulum*
Fracture of the femur*
Haemarthrosis
Hip dysplasia*
Luxation*
Septic arthritis
Traumatic arthritis*

Stifle
Caudal cruciate ligament rupture or avulsion
Cranial cruciate ligament rupture or avulsion*
Femorotibial luxation
Fracture of the femur*
Fracture of the fibula*
Fracture of the patella*
Fracture of the tibia*
Genu valgum

Haemarthrosis
Long digital extensor tendon avulsion
Meniscal trauma*
Osteochondrosis*
Patellar ligament rupture or avulsion
Patellar luxation*
Septic arthritis
Stifle hyperextension
Traumatic arthritis*

Hock

Calcaneal tendon rupture, laceration or avulsion
Collateral ligament avulsion
Congenital tarsal anomalies
Fracture of the tibia*
Fracture of the fibula*
Fractures of the metatarsal bones*
Fractures of the tarsal bones*
Gastrocnemius tendon rupture, laceration or avulsion
Growth plate disorders
Haemarthrosis
Luxation
Osteochondrosis*
Septic arthritis
Shearing injury
Tibial dysplasia
Traumatic arthritis*

Foot

Avulsion of the superficial or deep digital flexor tendon
Claw disease *q.v.*
Degenerative joint disease*
Fractures of the distal metatarsal bones*
Fractures of the phalanges*
Fractures of the sesamoid bones
Haemarthrosis
Injury to the integument*, e.g.
- Bite wound
- Foreign body
- Laceration

Other pathology of the integument*
Luxation
Septic arthritis
Sesamoid disease
Traumatic arthritis*

ADULT ANIMALS

Any site
Infection
Trauma
  - Bruising or strain of soft tissues
  - Laceration
  - Penetrating wound

Hip
Avascular necrosis of the femoral head*
Degenerative joint disease*
Fracture of the acetabulum*
Fracture of the femur*
Haemarthrosis
Hip dysplasia*
Luxation*
Myositis ossificans
Neoplasia*
  - Bone
  - Soft tissue
  - Metastatic
Septic arthritis
Traumatic arthritis*

Stifle
Caudal cruciate ligament rupture or avulsion
Cranial cruciate ligament rupture or avulsion*
Degenerative joint disease*
Femorotibial luxation
Fracture of the femur*
Fracture of the fibula*
Fracture of the patella*
Fracture of the tibia*
Haemarthrosis

Long digital extensor tendon avulsion
Meniscal trauma*
Neoplasia*
- Bone
- Soft tissue
- Metastatic
Osteochondrosis*
Patellar ligament rupture or avulsion
Patellar luxation*
Septic arthritis
Stifle hyperextension
Traumatic arthritis*

Hock

Calcaneal tendon rupture, laceration or avulsion
Collateral ligament avulsion
Degenerative joint disease*
Fracture of the fibula*
Fracture of the tibia*
Fractures of the metatarsal bones*
Fractures of the tarsal bones*
Gastrocnemius tendon rupture, laceration or avulsion
Growth plate disorders
Haemarthrosis
Luxation
Neoplasia*
- Bone
- Soft tissue
- Metastatic
Osteochondrosis*
Septic arthritis
Shearing injury
Superficial digital flexor luxation
Tibial dysplasia
Traumatic arthritis*

Foot

Avulsion of the superficial or deep digital flexor tendon
Claw disease* *q.v.*
Degenerative joint disease*

Fractures of distal metatarsal bones*
Fractures of phalanges*
Fractures of sesamoid bones
Haemarthrosis
Injury to the integument*, e.g.
- Bite wound
- Foreign body
- Laceration

Other pathology of the integument*
Luxation*
Neoplasia*
- Bone
- Soft tissue
- Metastatic

Septic arthritis
Sesamoid disease
Traumatic arthritis*
Traumatic tenosynovitis

1.7.3 Multiple joint/limb lameness

Young animals

Borreliosis
Chondrodysplasia
Drug reaction
- Sulphonamide
- Vaccine

Excessive joint laxity
- Collagen defect
- Dietary
- Traumatic

Haemarthroses
Metaphyseal osteopathy (D)
Nutritional secondary hyperthyroidism
Panosteitis
Polyarthritis
Osteochondrosis*
Septic arthritis
Viral arthritis

Adult animals

Borreliosis
Chondrodysplasia
Degenerative joint disease*
Drug reaction
- Sulphonamide
- Vaccine

Excessive joint laxity
- Collagen defect
- Dietary
- Traumatic

Haemarthroses
Hyperparathyroidism
Neuromuscular disease
Osteochondrosis*
Nutritional, e.g.
- Hypervitaminosis A
- Copper deficiency

Periosteal proliferative arthritis
Polyarthritis
Septic arthritis
Systemic lupus erythematosus
Viral arthritis

1.8 Reproductive historical signs

1.8.1 Failure to observe oestrus

Abnormal sex chromosomes
Early embryonic death *q.v.*
Idiopathic
Immune-mediated oophoritis
Inadequate display of oestrus*
Inadequate observation of oestrus*
Inappropriate photoperiod (C)
Lactational anoestrus*
Panhypopituitarism

Physical/athletic training
Poor diet
Prepuberty*
Previous ovariectomy*
Pseudohermaphroditism
Pseudopregnancy*
Seasonal anoestrus (C)*
Social factors
Spontaneous ovulation
Sterile matings
True hermaphroditism

Concurrent disease

Hyperadrenocorticism
Hypoadrenocorticism (D)
Hypothyroidism* (D)
Poor body condition

Iatrogenic

Anabolic steroids
Androgens
Glucocorticoids
Progesterones

Ovarian disease

Ovarian aplasia
Ovarian cysts and tumours
- Granulosa–thecal cell tumours
- Luteal cysts
- Other neoplasms or cysts causing ovarian atrophy

Ovarian hypoplasia
Senile ovarian failure

Stress*

Frequent showing
Frequent travel
Overcrowding
Temperature extremes

1.8.2   Irregular seasons

Short pro-oestrus followed by anoestrus

Poor diet
Shortened inter-pro-oestrus intervals (see succeeding text)
Stress

Reduced intensity of visible signs of oestrus

Concurrent disease*
Drugs*
- Anabolic steroids
- Androgens
- Glucocorticoids
- Progesterones

Persistence of oestrus behaviour

Signs of oestrus in the absence of true hormonal oestrus

Vaginal foreign body
Vaginal tumour
Vaginitis*
Vulvitis*

Prolonged pro-oestrus/oestrus

Excessive adrenal production of oestrogen (C)
Follicular cysts*
Hepatic disease
Merging of waves of follicular growth (C)
Normal in young females*

Iatrogenic

Drugs used to prevent pregnancy after mating
Exogenous gonadotrophins

Ovarian tumours

Adenocarcinoma
Cystadenoma
Granulosa cell tumour

Shortened inter-pro-oestrus interval

Follicular cysts
Frequent episodes of pro-oestrus
Ovulatory failure
Short anoestrus
Split heats

Iatrogenic

Bromocriptine
Cabergoline
Prostaglandins

Prolonged inter-pro-oestrus interval

Normal in some breeds
Hypothyroidism* (D)
Idiopathic
Ovarian cysts or neoplasia
Severe systemic disease
Silent heat

1.8.3 Infertility in the female with normal oestrus

Failure to achieve intromission

Male factors* *q.v.*

Congenital defects of the vestibule and vagina

Intersexes
Vaginal septa
Vestibulovaginal strictures
Vulval constrictions

Acquired vaginal conditions

Foreign body
Post-partum fibrosis
Transmissible venereal tumour
Vaginal hyperplasia*

Vaginal tumours
Vaginal ulceration

Failure of ovulation
Idiopathic (D)
Inadequate number of matings (C)
Incorrect timing of mating* (C)

Miscellaneous
Cervical stenosis
Cystic endometrial hyperplasia*
Early embryonic loss *q.v.*
Endometritis
Herpesvirus
Hypoluteodism/insufficient progesterone secretion by corpus luteum
Incorrect timing of mating/insemination*
Infertile male
Non-patent oviducts or uterus
Segmental aplasia of the paramesonephric (Müllerian) duct
Stress
Uterine polyps
Uterine tumours

1.8.4   Male infertility

Failure to achieve intromission
Female factors *q.v.*

Acquired abnormalities
Neoplasia of the penis/prepuce
Phimosis
Trauma of the penis/prepuce
Urethral obstruction and subsequent haematoma

Congenital abnormalities, e.g.
Diphallus
Penile hypoplasia
Persistent penile frenulum
Preputial stenosis
Pseudohermaphroditism

Miscellaneous
Incomplete erection
Ineffective thrusting
- Experience*
- Poor socialisation*
- Short os penis
- Size discrepancy*
- Trauma (desensitised glans)
Premature full attainment of erection in inexperienced dog*
Premature loss of erection*

Inability to mount the female
Prostatic disease *q.v.*
Orthopaedic disease*

Lack of fertility where normal mating(s) is(are) achieved
Failure of/incomplete ejaculation
Discomfort or stress during mating*
Inadequate tie*
Retrograde ejaculation
- Disorder of the sympathetic nervous system
- Urethral sphincter incompetence

Lack of libido
Age related
Prepubertal*
Senility*

Behavioural
Inexperience*
Previous bad experience when mating*
Training not to display sexual interest*

Concurrent/systemic disease*, e.g.
Hypoadrenocorticism
Hypogonadism
Hypothyroidism* (D)

Diet
Malnutrition
Obesity*

Drugs
> Anabolic steroids
> Cimetidine
> Glucocorticoids
> Ketoconazole
> Oestrogens
> Overuse of testosterone
> Progestagens

Management
> Overuse*

Testicular disease
> Idiopathic testicular degeneration
> Orchitis
> Sertoli cell tumour

Low/absent sperm number or quality

Artefact
> Poor collection technique/analysis*

Acquired defects
> Infections causing azoospermia or abnormal sperm/semen
> - Balanoposthitis
> - Epididymitis
> - Orchitis
> - Prostatitis
> - Urethritis
>
> Increases in testicular temperature
> - Chemotherapeutics, e.g.
>   - Chlorambucil
>   - Cisplatin
>   - Cyclophosphamide
> - High environmental temperature
> - Hyperthermia
> - Iatrogenic
> - Orchitis in the contralateral testis
> - Other drugs
>   - Anabolic steroids
>   - Androgens
>   - Glucocorticoids

- Radiation therapy/excessive radiography
- Scrotal dermatitis

Local trauma
- Dog bites
- Kicks/blows
- Lacerations

Neoplasia of the testis
Overuse*
Pain*
Prepuberty*
Retrograde ejaculation
Toxins

Congenital defects

Cryptorchidism
Genetic abnormalities in spermatogenesis
- Chromosomal abnormalities, e.g.
  - XXY syndrome (D)
  - 38,XY/57,XXY (C)
- Immotile cilia (Kartagener's syndrome)

Segmental aplasia of the duct system
Testicular hypoplasia

1.8.5 Vaginal/vulval discharge

Ovarian remnant syndrome
Pseudopregnancy*
Pyometra*
Stump pyometra*
Vaginal or uterine neoplasia
Vaginitis*
Vulvitis*

1.8.6 Abortion

Drugs, e.g.

Cabergoline
Corticosteroids
Prostaglandins

Habitual abortion

Abnormal uterine environment, e.g.
* Cystic endometrial hyperplasia

Poor luteal function

Infection

Brucella canis (D)
Canine adenovirus (D)
Canine distemper virus (D)*
Canine herpesvirus (D)
Chlamydophila psittaci (C)
Ehrlichiosis
Feline herpesvirus (C)*
Feline infectious peritonitis (C)*
Feline leukaemia virus (C)*
Feline panleukopenia virus (C)*
Leishmaniasis
Toxoplasmosis

1.8.7　Dystocia

MATERNAL CAUSES

Obstruction of the birth canal

Congenital uterine malformations
* Aplasia of the cervix
* Aplasia of the corpus uteri
* Aplasia of the uterine horns

Fibrosis of the birth canal
Narrow pelvic canal
* Congenital
* Fracture*
* Immaturity*

Neoplasia
Uterine malposition
Uterine rupture

Uterine torsion
Vaginal septa

Uterine inertia*

Primary uterine inertia
Fatty infiltration of the myometrium
Hormonal deficiencies
Hypocalcaemia* *q.v.*
Inherited
Maternal systemic disease
Overstretching of the myometrium, e.g.
- Excessive intrauterine fluids
- Large foetuses*
- Large litter*

Poor diet
Senile changes*
Single puppy syndrome*

Secondary uterine inertia
Exhaustion of the myometrium*
- Obstruction of birth canal*
- Prolonged labour*

FOETAL CAUSES

Malpresentation*

Backward flexion of front legs
Breech
Lateral or downward deviation of the head
Posterior
Transverse
Two foetuses presenting simultaneously

Oversized foetuses

Physically normal but large puppy*
Monstrosities
- Duplications
- Hydrocephalus
- Oedema

1.8.8   Neonatal mortality

Congenital abnormalities*, e.g.
Congenital heart disease
Hydrocephalus
Hypothyroidism

Infections*, e.g.
Feline calicivirus*
Feline herpesvirus*
Feline infectious peritonitis*
Feline parvovirus*
Septicaemia

Maternal/management factors*
Asphyxiation
Euthanasia for reasons of congenital deformities or undesirable
cosmetic features
Hypoglycaemia *q.v.*, e.g.
  • Secondary to sepsis
Hypothermia
Inadequate lactation
Poor environment, e.g.
  • Draughts
  • Heating
Poor hygiene
Poor mothering
Poor nutrition/health of breeding stock

Miscellaneous
Fading puppy syndrome*
Low birth weight
Neonatal isoerythrolysis
Stillbirth

1.9   Urological historical signs

1.9.1   Pollakiuria/dysuria/stranguria

Normal urine
Behavioural*
Feline lower urinary tract disease
Idiopathic detrusor-urethral dyssynergia
Neuromuscular

With haematuria, pyuria or bacteriuria
Diabetes mellitus*
Feline lower urinary tract disease* (C)
Hyperadrenocorticism/corticosteroid treatment
Iatrogenic disorders
Infection
Infiltrative urethral diseases
Neoplasia
Neuromuscular disorders
Prostatic disease
Renal disease* *q.v.*
Structural abnormalities
Trauma/bladder rupture
Urolithiasis*

1.9.2   Polyuria/polydipsia (see Section 1.1.1 for full differentials)

Diet
Drugs/toxins
Congenital lack of ADH receptors
Electrolyte disorders
Endocrine disease
Hepatobiliary disease
Hypothalamic disease
Infectious disease

Metabolic (e.g. hypercalcaemia)
Neoplasia*
Pericardial effusion
Physiological
Polycythaemia
Psychogenic
Renal disorders

1.9.3   Anuria/oliguria

Pre-renal
Dehydration*
Hypoadrenocorticism (D)
Shock *q.v.**

Renal
Acute kidney injury *q.v.*
Chronic kidney disease*

Post-renal
Prostatic disease*
Urethral spasm

Neoplasia
Bladder
Extra-urinary tract
Urethra

Trauma
Avulsion of ureters
Ruptured bladder/urethra

*Urolithiasis**
Nephroliths
Ureteroliths
Uroliths in the bladder or urethra

1.9.4   Haematuria

Extra-urogenital disease
Coagulopathy *q.v.*
Drugs/toxins
  • Paracetamol
Heatstroke
Thrombocytopenia/thrombocytopathia

Penile disease
Neoplasia
Trauma

Physiological
Pro-oestrus

Prostatic disease
Abscess
Benign prostatic hyperplasia* (D)
Cysts
Neoplasia
Prostatitis*

Pseudohaematuria (non-haematuria-related red urine)
Bilirubinuria *q.v.*
Food pigments
  • Blackberries
  • Beets
  • Rhubarb
Haemoglobinuria *q.v.*
Myoglobinuria *q.v.*
Phenazopyridine
Phenolphthalein
Phenothiazines

Renal disease
Cysts
Glomerulonephritis

Iatrogenic
* Biopsy
* Fine-needle aspirate

Idiopathic renal haematuria

Infarction, e.g.
* Disseminated intravascular coagulation

Neoplasia*

Parasites
* *Dioctophyma renale*

Pyelonephritis

Renal telangiectasia

Trauma

Uroliths*

Ureteral, urinary bladder and urethral disease

Drugs
* Cyclophosphamide

Feline lower urinary tract disease*

Iatrogenic
* Cystocentesis*
* Forceful catheterisation*

Neoplasia

Parasites
* *Capillaria plica*

Polyps

Trauma*

Urethritis

Uroliths*

Uterine disease

Metritis

Neoplasia

Pyometra*

Sub-involution*

Vaginal disease

Neoplasia

Trauma

1.9.5 Urinary incontinence/inappropriate urination

With bladder distension

Detrusor atony
Bladder over-distension
Dysautonomia
Lower motor neurone disease
Neoplastic infiltration of the bladder wall
Upper motor neurone disease

Functional obstruction
Reflex dyssynergia*
Upper motor neurone disease
Urethral inflammation*
Urethral pain

Partial physical obstruction
Granulomatous urethritis
Neoplasia
Prostatic disease*
Retroflexion of the bladder into a perineal hernia
Urethral fibrosis/stricture
Urolithiasis*
Vestibulovaginal stenosis

Without bladder distension

Bladder hypercontractility
Chronic partial obstruction*
Detrusor instability
Inflammation*
Neoplasia

Miscellaneous
Behavioural
Ectopic ureters

Iatrogenic
  • Ureterovaginal fistulation
Secondary to polydipsia/polyuria
Ureterocoele
Urolithiasis

Reduced bladder storage
  Fibrosis
  Hypoplasia
  Neoplasia

Urethral sphincter incompetence
  Congenital
  Hormone responsive*
  Intersex
  Prostatic disease*
  Urethral inflammation*
  Urethral neoplasia
  Urinary tract infection*

PART 2
PHYSICAL SIGNS

2.1 General/miscellaneous physical signs

2.1.1 Abnormalities of body temperature – hyperthermia

TRUE FEVER

Drugs/toxins
Adder bites
Amphotericin B
Aspirin
Benzalkonium chloride
Benzodiazepines
Borax
Cannabis
Carbamate
Daffodil
Dichlorophen
Diclofenac sodium
Dinoprost tromethamine
Glyphosate
Horse chestnut
Hymenoptera stings
Indomethacin
Ivermectin

Differential Diagnosis in Small Animal Medicine, Second Edition.
Alex Gough and Kate Murphy.
© 2015 John Wiley & Sons, Ltd. Published 2015 by John Wiley & Sons, Ltd.

Metaldehyde
Organophosphates
Oxytetracycline
Paracetamol
Paraquat
Penicillamine
Petroleum distillates
Phenytoin
Poinsettia
Procainamide
Pyrethrin/pyrethroids
Salbutamol
Theobromine
Yew

Immune-mediated disease

Autoimmune skin disease
- Bullous pemphigoid
- Discoid lupus erythematosus
- Pemphigus erythematosus
- Pemphigus foliaceus
- Pemphigus vulgaris

Drug reactions
Evan syndrome
Familial renal amyloidosis (Shar Pei fever)
Immune-mediated haemolytic anaemia*
Immune-mediated joint disease*
- Erosive
  - Rheumatoid arthritis
- Non-erosive
  - Chronic inflammatory/infectious
  - Idiopathic
  - Enteropathic
  - Neoplasia
  - Periosteal proliferative arthritis
  - Systemic lupus erythematosus

Immune-mediated thrombocytopenia
Lymphadenitis
Pemphigus
Plasmacytic-lymphocytic gonitis

Polyarteritis nodosa
Polymyositis
Steroid-responsive meningitis
Systemic lupus erythematosus

Immunodeficiency syndromes

Defects in specific immunity, e.g.
Agammaglobulinaemia
C3 deficiency
Canine leucocyte adhesion deficiency
Lethal acrodermatitis
Low immunoglobulins in Weimaraners (D)
Neutrophil defect of Weimaraners (D)
Pneumocystic pneumonia in miniature
Dachshunds (D)
Transient hypogammaglobulinaemia
Selective immunoglobulin (IgA) deficiency
Selective IgM deficiency
Severe combined immunodeficiency disease

Defects in non-specific immunity
Bone marrow dyscrasia in Poodles (D)
Canine cyclic haematopoiesis (D)
Canine granulocytopathy syndrome (D)
Chediak–Higashi syndrome (C)
Complement deficiency (D)
Hypotrichosis with thymic aplasia (C)
Immotile cilia syndrome
Trapped neutrophil syndrome
Pelger–Huet anomaly

Secondary immunodeficiencies
Drugs
 • Corticosteroids
 • Immunosuppressive therapy
Endocrine
 • Hyperadrenocorticism
Infectious, e.g.
 • Canine distemper virus* (D)
 • Demodecosis*

- Feline immunodeficiency syndrome* (C)
- Feline leukaemia virus* (C)
- Parvovirus

Metabolic
- Uraemia

Neoplastic
- Haematopoietic

Nutritional
- Zinc deficiency

Infection

Bacterial

Generalised/multifocal, e.g.
- Bartonellosis
- Brucellosis (D)
- Leptospirosis*
- Lyme disease
- *Mycobacterium* spp.
- *Mycoplasma* spp.
- Plague
- Septicaemia from septic focus

Localised, e.g.
- Abscess*, e.g.
  - Dental
  - Lung
  - Retrobulbar
- Cellulitis*
- Cholangiohepatitis
- Cystitis
- Dental disease*
- Discospondylitis
- Endocarditis
- Gastrointestinal infection*
- Mastitis
- Metritis*
- Osteomyelitis*
- Peritonitis*
- Pneumonia*
- Prostatitis*

- Pyelonephritis
- Pyometra/stump pyometra*
- Pyothorax*
- Septic arthritis*
- Urinary tract infection*

Fungal, e.g.
Aspergillosis
Blastomycosis
Coccidioidomycosis
Cryptococcosis
Histoplasmosis

Parasitic, e.g.
Aberrant helminth migration
Babesiosis
Chagas disease (Trypanosomiasis)
Cytauxzoon felis
Dirofilaria immitis
Hepatozoonosis
Leishmaniasis

Protozoal, e.g.
Neosporosis (D)
Toxoplasmosis

Rickettsial, e.g.
Ehrlichiosis
Rocky Mountain spotted fever (D)
Salmon poisoning

Viral (many), e.g.
Canine distemper virus* (D)
Canine hepatitis virus* (D)
Canine parainfluenza virus* (D)
Canine parvovirus* (D)
Feline calicivirus* (C)
Feline herpes virus* (C)
Feline immunodeficiency virus* (C)
Feline infectious peritonitis* (C)
Feline leukaemia virus* (C)
Feline panleukopenia virus* (C)

Miscellaneous

Metabolic bone disorders
- Hypervitaminosis A (C)
- Metaphyseal osteopathy
- Nutritional secondary hyperthyroidism
- Panosteitis

Pansteatitis (C)

Portosystemic shunt

True pyrexia of unknown origin

Neoplasia

Lymphoma*

Lymphoproliferative disease

Leukaemia

Histiocytic disease (systemic histiocytosis, malignant histiocytosis, histiocytic sarcoma)

Myeloproliferative disease

Solid tumours*

Tissue damage*

Surgery*

Trauma*

OTHER CAUSES OF HYPERTHERMIA

Heat stroke*

Hyperpyrexic syndrome

Increased muscular activity

Episodic myokymia

Hypocalcaemic tetany *q.v.*

Normal exercise*

Pain

Seizures* *q.v.*

Stress

Pathological hyperthermia

Hypermetabolic states
- Hyperthyroidism* (C)
- Pheochromocytoma

Hypothalamic lesions

Malignant hyperthermia

2.1.2 Abnormalities of body temperature – hypothermia

Drugs/toxins

Alphachloralose
Baclofen
Benzodiazepines
Cannabis
Daffodil
Ethylene glycol
General anaesthetics
Ivermectin
Loperamide
Paracetamol
Sedatives
Yew

Miscellaneous

Aortic thromboembolism* (C)
Cardiac disease* *q.v.*
Coma *q.v.*
Environmental cold*
Hypoadrenocorticism (D)
Hypothalamic disorders
Hypothyroidism* (D)
Loss of thermoregulatory abilities following heat stroke
Near drowning
Severe sepsis/endotoxaemia*

2.1.3 Enlarged lymph nodes

INFILTRATION

Neoplastic disease

Haemolymphatic
Leukaemia
Lymphoma*
Lymphomatoid granulomatosis

Malignant histiocytosis
Multiple myeloma
Systemic mastocytosis

Metastatic
Adenocarcinoma
Carcinoma
Malignant melanoma
Mast cell tumour
Sarcoma

Non-neoplastic disease
Eosinophilic granuloma complex
Mast cell infiltration

PROLIFERATION/INFLAMMATION
Infectious
Algal
Prototheocosis

Bacterial
Actinomycosis
Bartonella spp.
Brucella canis (D)
Corynebacterium spp.
Localised infection
Mycobacterium spp.
Nocardiosis
Septicaemia
Streptococcus spp.
Yersinia pestis

Fungal
Aspergillosis
Blastomycosis
Coccidioidomycosis
Cryptococcosis
Histoplasmosis

Phycomycosis
Sporotrichosis

Parasitic
Babesiosis
Cytauxzoonosis
Demodecosis
Hepatozoonosis
Leishmaniasis
Trypanosomiasis

Protozoal
Neosporosis (D)
Toxoplasmosis

Rickettsial
Ehrlichiosis
Rocky Mountain spotted fever
Salmon poisoning

Viral
Canine herpes virus* (D)
Feline immunodeficiency virus* (C)
Feline infectious peritonitis* (C)
Feline leukaemia virus* (C)
Infectious canine hepatitis* (D)

Non-infectious
Dermatopathic lymphadenopathy
Drug reactions
Idiopathic
Immune-mediated
- Immune-mediated polyarthritides
- Mineral-associated lymphadenopathy
- Granulomatous lymphadenitis
- Puppy strangles* (D)
- Rheumatoid arthritis
- Systemic lupus erythematosus
Localised inflammation*
Post-vaccine

2.1.4   Diffuse pain

Gastrointestinal disease, e.g.

Cholecystolithiasis/cholecystitis*
Gastrointestinal inflammation/ulceration
Gastrointestinal parasitism*
Pancreatitis*

Miscellaneous
Panniculitis

MUSCULOSKELETAL DISEASE, E.G.

Polyarthritis
Polymyositis

Neurological disease, e.g.

Meningoencephalitis
Spinal disease* *q.v.*
Thalamic pain syndrome

Urological disease, e.g.

Cystitis
Prostatic disease*
Pyelonephritis
Renal parasitism
Urethral tumour
Urolithiasis

Other causes of abdominal pain q.v.

Mesenteric thrombosis
Pansteatitis
Peritonitis

2.1.5   Peripheral oedema

Generalised

Hypoalbuminaemia* *q.v.*
Increased central venous pressure

- Central venous occlusion
  - Neoplasia
  - Thro mbosis
- Congestive heart failure*

Vasculitis

Localised

Arteriovenous fistula
Cellulitis*
Drugs/toxins
- Alphaxalone/alphadolone
- Paracetamol
- Salbutamol

Inflammation*
Lymphangitis
Lymphoedema
Neurogenic or hormonal vasoactive stimuli
Proximal venous obstruction
Vascular trauma
Vasculitis

Regional

Bilateral forelimb oedema/head and neck oedema
Cranial vena cava syndrome
- Compression of cranial vena cava,
  e.g. by mediastinal mass
- Granuloma of cranial vena cava
- Neoplasia of cranial vena cava
- Thrombosis of cranial vena cava

Bilateral hind limb oedema
Budd–Chiari-like syndrome
Obstruction of sublumbar lymph nodes,
e.g. neoplasia

Increased central venous pressure
Central lymph obstruction
Central venous occlusion, e.g.
- Mediastinal mass
- Thrombosis

2.1.6 Hypertension

Adrenal disease
Hyperadrenocorticism
Hyperaldosteronism
Pheochromocytoma

Anaemia* q.v.

CNS disease q.v.

Drugs/toxins
Corticosteroids
Ciclosporin A
Dobutamine
Dopamine
Doxapram
Erythropoietin
Fludrocortisone
Phenylpropanolamine
Theobromine

Endocrine disease
Acromegaly
Diabetes mellitus* (D)
Hyperoestrogenism
Hyperthyroidism* (C)

Hyperviscosity
Hyperglobulinaemia *q.v.*
Polycythaemia *q.v.*

Iatrogenic
Overzealous fluid administration

Idiopathic
Essential/primary hypertension

Renal disease
Renal arterial disease

Renal parenchymal disease
- Amyloidosis
- Chronic interstitial nephritis*
- Glomerulonephritis
- Glomerulosclerosis
- Pyelonephritis

Thyroid disease

Hyperthyroidism* (C)

2.1.7 Hypotension

Decreased cardiac function

Arrhythmias* *q.v.*
Cardiomyopathy*
Congenital heart disease
Electrolyte/acid–base disorders* *q.v.*
Hypoxia
Valvular disease*

Decreased preload

Heatstroke*
Hypoadrenocorticism (D)
Hypovolaemia*
- Blood donation
- Burns
- Effusions *q.v.*
- Diarrhoea *q.v.*
- Haemorrhage *q.v.*
- Polyuria without polydipsia *q.v.*
- Vomiting *q.v.*

Decreased vascular tone

Anaphylaxis
Babesiosis
Electrolyte/acid–base disorders* *q.v.*
Hypoxia
Neurological disease *q.v.*
Systemic inflammatory response syndrome

Decreased venous return

Cardiac tamponade
Caval syndrome/heartworm disease
Gastric dilatation/volvulus*
Pneumothorax* *q.v.*
Positive pressure ventilation
Restrictive pericarditis

Drugs/toxins

ACE inhibitors
Adder bites
Amiloride
Amiodarone
Daffodil
Diazoxide
Dopamine
General anaesthetics and sedatives
Hydralazine
Hymenoptera stings
Indomethacin
Isosorbide dinitrate
Lignocaine
Medetomidine
Mexiletine
Midazolam
Mistletoe
Nitroprusside
Oxytetracycline (intravenous)
Phenoxybenzamine
Prazosin
Procainamide
Propofol
Pyridostigmine
Quinidine
Ranitidine (intravenous)
Rhododendron
Snake venom
Sotalol
Terbutaline
Terfenadine

Tricyclic antidepressants
Verapamil
Xylazine
Yew

2.2 Gastrointestinal/abdominal physical signs

2.2.1 Oral lesions

Congenital deformities e.g.
Cleft palate

Neoplasia

Oropharyngeal tumours
Extramedullary plasmacytoma
Fibroma/fibrosarcoma
Fibropapilloma
Granular cell tumour
Haemangiosarcoma
Histiocytoma
Lymphoma
Mast cell tumour
Melanoma*
Mixed mesenchymal sarcoma
Papilloma (D)
Rhabdomyosarcoma
Squamous cell carcinoma
Transmissible venereal tumour (D)

Odontogenic tumours
Acanthomatous epulides
Ameloblastic adenomatoid
Ameloblastoma
Calcifying epithelial odontogenic tumour
Cementoma
Dentinoma

Fibromatous epulides
Fibromyxoma
Hamartoma
Inductive fibroameloblastoma (C)
Keratinising ameloblastoma (C)
Odontogenic fibroma
Odontoma
Ossifying epulides

Inflammatory masses, e.g.
Feline eosinophilic granuloma complex*

Oral ulceration
Immune-mediated/inflammatory, e.g.
- Eosinophilic granuloma complex*
- Lymphoplasmacytic*

Infectious, e.g.
- Feline calicivirus

Ingestion of irritant/caustic substances*
Metabolic, e.g.
- Uraemia* *q.v.*

Traumatic*

Periodontitis/gingivitis
Bacterial infection*
Diabetes mellitus*
Diet (non-abrasive)*
Immune deficiency, e.g.
- Feline immunodeficiency virus* (C)
- Feline leukaemia virus* (C)

Immune-mediated disease, e.g.
- Lymphoplasmacytic*

Periodontal foreign material*, e.g.
- Grass
- Hair

Tooth abnormalities*, e.g.
- Crowding
- Malocclusion
- Rough surfaces

Salivary gland enlargement

Infarction
Infection
Neoplasia
- Acinic cell tumour
- Adenocarcinoma
- Monomorphic adenoma
- Mucoepidermoid tumour
- Pleomorphic adenoma
- Undifferentiated carcinoma

Sialadenitis
Sialadenosis
Sialocele

Stomatitis

Immune-mediated/inflammatory, e.g.
- Eosinophilic stomatitis
- Lymphoplasmacytic stomatitis*

Infection, e.g.
- *Bartonella henselae*
- Feline calicivirus* (C)
- Feline herpes virus* (C)

Ingestion of irritant/caustic substances
Metabolic, e.g. uraemia*
Traumatic*

Tooth disease

Caries
Feline odontoclastic resorptive lesions* (C)
Trauma*

2.2.2 Abdominal distension

Abdominal neoplasia*
Ascites* *q.v.*
Bladder distension* *q.v.*
Gastric dilatation*
Gastric distension*
Intestinal dilatation/volvulus

Obesity
Obstipation* *q.v.*
Organomegaly*
- Enlarged kidney *q.v.*
- Enlarged uterus *q.v.*
- Hepatomegaly *q.v.*
- Splenomegaly *q.v.*

Pneumoperitoneum
Pregnancy
Weakness of abdominal musculature
- Hyperadrenocorticism
- Ruptured prepubic tendon

2.2.3 Abdominal pain

Drugs/toxins

Allopurinol
Blue-green algae
Borax
Daffodil
Diclofenac sodium
Dieffenbachia
Horse chestnut
Ibuprofen
Indomethacin
Itraconazole
Loperamide
Metaldehyde
Misoprostol
Naproxen
NPK fertilisers
Paracetamol
Paraquat
Petroleum distillates
Phenoxy acid herbicides
Poinsettia
Rhododendron
Theobromine
Zinc sulphate

Gastrointestinal disease
Colitis*
Constipation* *q.v.*
Enteritis*
Gastric dilatation/volvulus* (D)
Gastric foreign body*
Gastric ulceration*
Gastritis*
Intestinal volvulus
Neoplasia*
Small intestinal foreign body*

Hepatobiliary disease
Cholangitis
Cholecystitis*
Cholelithiasis
Gall bladder obstruction
Hepatitis*
Liver lobe torsion
Portal hypertension

Mechanical factors
Dilatation of a hollow viscus
Bladder distension* *q.v.*
Gastric dilatation/volvulus* (D)
Intestinal dilatation, e.g.
- Foreign body
- Volvulus

Obstruction of outflow
Obstruction of bile outflow
Urinary tract obstruction

Mesenteric tension/traction/torsion
Abscess
Bowel incarceration in hernia or mesenteric tear
Cryptorchid testicular torsion
Foreign body*
Haematoma
Intestinal volvulus

Gastric dilatation/volvulus* (D)
Intussusception*
Neoplasia
Splenic torsion
Stenosis/stricture
Uterine torsion

Miscellaneous

Mesenteric thromboembolism
Sterile nodular panniculitis and pansteatitis
in Weimaraners

Musculoskeletal pain

Abdominal muscle rupture
Referred spinal pain*

Organ rupture

Bile duct
Gall bladder
Intestine
Spleen
Stomach
Urinary tract
Uterus, e.g.
  • Pyometra

Pancreas

Pancreatic abscess
Pancreatitis*
Pancreatic neoplasia

Peritoneal cavity

Ascites *q.v.*
Pneumoperitoneum

Haemoabdomen
  Angiostrongylus vasorum infection
  Coagulopathy *q.v.*
  Neoplasia*
  Trauma*

Peritonitis
  Blunt trauma*
  Feline infectious peritonitis* (C)
  Iatrogenic, e.g.
    • Post-surgical*
  Pancreatitis*
  Penetrating trauma
  Primary (C)
  Prostatitis*
  Rupture or penetration of gastrointestinal tract
  Ruptured pyometra

Uroabdomen
  Rupture of urinary tract

Reproductive system
  Labour/dystocia*
  Metritis*
  Prostatic disease
  Pyometra*

Trauma
  Fractures*
  Ruptured viscus

Urinary system
  Cystitis*
  Lower urinary tract obstruction*
  Nephritis
  Nephrolithiasis
  Pyelonephritis
  Ureteral obstruction

2.2.4 Perianal swelling

*Anal/rectal prolapse**
  Faecal tenesmus*

Anal sac disease
  Anal sac abscess*
  Anal sac adenocarcinoma

Anal sac impaction*
Anal sacculitis*

Neoplasia
Perianal adenoma*
Other perianal neoplasia

*Perineal hernia**
Idiopathic
Secondary to causes of tenesmus *q.v.*

2.2.5 Jaundice

PRE-HEPATIC
Haemolytic anaemia *q.v.*
Congenital porphyria
Ineffective erythropoiesis
Internal haemorrhage
Severe myolysis

HEPATIC

Drugs/toxins
Barbiturates
Blue-green algae
Carbimazole
Diazepam
Glipizide
Glucocorticoids
Glyphosate
Griseofulvin
Ketoconazole
Methimazole
Methyltestosterone
Metronidazole
Mexiletine
NSAIDS, e.g.
  • Carprofen

- Ibuprofen
- Paracetamol
- Phenylbutazone

Phenobarbitone
Plastic explosives
Primidone
Salicylates
Sulphasalazine
Tetracycline

Intrahepatic cholestasis

Hepatic necrosis, e.g.
   Infection
   Toxin

Infection
   Bacterial*
   Fungal
   Viral
   - Adenovirus* (D)
   - Feline immunodeficiency virus* (C)
   - Feline infectious peritonitis* (C)
   - Feline leukaemia virus* (C)

Inflammation
   Cholangitis/cholangiohepatitis*

Miscellaneous
   Amyloidosis
   Cirrhosis
   Hepatic erythrohaemophagic syndrome
   Hepatic lipidosis
   Polycystic kidney disease with
   liver cysts (C)

Neoplasia, e.g.
   Lymphoma*
   Mast cell tumour
   Myeloproliferative disease

POST-HEPATIC

Bile duct occlusion

Extraluminal
Choledochal cysts (C)
Duodenal disease
Pancreatic neoplasia
Pancreatitis*
Polycystic disease (C)
Secondary to peribiliary disease
Stricture at *porta hepatis*

Intramural
Cholangitis
Cholecystitis*
Choledochitis
Gall bladder/duct neoplasia

Intraluminal
Choledochal cysts (C)
Cholelithiasis
Gall bladder mucocoele
Haemobilia
Inspissated bile
Polycystic kidney disease with liver cysts(C)

2.2.6   Abnormal liver palpation

Generalised enlargement

Drugs
Glucocorticoids

Endocrine disease
Diabetes mellitus*
Hyperadrenocorticism

Inflammation/infection, e.g.
Abscess*
Cholangiohepatitis*
Feline infectious peritonitis* (C)

Fungal infection
Granuloma
Hepatitis*
Lymphocytic cholangitis

Miscellaneous
Amyloidosis
Cholestasis (see Jaundice *q.v.*)
Cirrhosis (early)
Hepatic lipidosis
Nodular hyperplasia
Peliosis
Storage diseases

Neoplasia * *e.g.*
Lymphoma
Malignant histiocytosis

Venous congestion
Caudal vena cava occlusion (post-caval syndrome)
- Adhesions
- Cardiac neoplasia
- Congenital cardiac disease
- Diaphragmatic rupture/hernia*
- Dirofilariasis
- Pericardial disease
- Thoracic mass*
- Thrombosis
- Trauma
Right-sided congestive heart failure, e.g.
- Dilated cardiomyopathy*
- Pericardial effusion

Focal enlargement
Abscess*
Biliary pseudocyst
Cyst
Granuloma
Haematoma*
Hepatic arteriovenous fistula
Hyperplastic/regenerative nodule*
Liver lobe torsion

Neoplasia
   Adenocarcinoma*
   Biliary cystadenoma
   Haemangiosarcoma*
   Hepatocellular carcinoma*
   Hepatoma
   Lymphoma*
   Malignant histiocytosis
   Metastatic*

Reduced liver size
   Cirrhosis*
   Diaphragmatic rupture/hernia* (apparent reduction)
   Hypoadrenocorticism (D)
   Idiopathic hepatic fibrosis
   Portosystemic shunt
     • Acquired
     • Congenital

2.3   Cardiorespiratory physical signs

2.3.1   Dyspnoea/tachypnoea

Drugs/toxins
   Benzalkonium chloride
   Blue-green algae
   Dichlorophen
   Ibuprofen
   Metaldehyde
   Naproxen
   Paracetamol (methaemoglobinaemia)
   Paraquat
   Salbutamol
   Strychnine
   Terfenadine

Physiological causes
   Exercise
   Fear

High ambient temperature
Pain

Upper airway disorders

Cervical tracheal disease
   Extraluminal compression
   Foreign body
   Hypoplasia/stenosis
   Neoplasia
   • Extraluminal
   • Intraluminal
      Adenocarcinoma
      Chondroma
      Chondrosarcoma
      Leiomyoma
      Lymphoma
      Osteochondroma
      Osteosarcoma
      Plasmacytoma
      Polyps
      Rhabdomyosarcoma
      Squamous cell carcinoma
   Tracheal collapse*
   Trauma

Laryngeal disease
   Everted saccules* (D)
   Inflammation
   Laryngeal paralysis* (D)
   Neoplasia
   Oedema*

Nasal disease (more often dyspnoea than tachypnoea) e.g.
   Aspergillosis
   Foreign body*
   Inflammatory disease*
   Nasopharyngeal polyp
   Neoplasia
   Stenotic nares

Pharyngeal disease
Elongated or oedematous soft palate* (D)
Enlarged tonsils*

Lower airway disorders

Thoracic tracheal disease, e.g.
Extraluminal compression
Foreign body
Hypoplasia/stenosis
Neoplasia (extra- or intraluminal)
Tracheal collapse*
Trauma

Bronchial disease
Bronchiectasis
Broncho-oesophageal fistula
Bronchitis* (D)
Cystic-bullous lung disease, e.g. secondary to emphysema
Eosinophilic bronchitis*
Extraluminal compression
  • Enlarged left atrium
  • Hilar lymphadenopathy, e.g.
    ◦ Fungal disease
    ◦ Granulomatous disease
    ◦ Neoplasia
Feline asthma* (C)
Foreign body
Lungworm
Neoplasia
Primary ciliary dyskinesia

Pulmonary parenchymal disease
Foreign body
Abscess
Chronic pulmonary fibrosis
Eosinophilic bronchopneumonopathy
Eosinophilic pneumonitis
Eosinophilic pulmonary granulomatosis
Hilar lymph node enlargement
Inhalation pneumonia
Idiopathic pulmonary fibrosis

Inflammatory disease
Irritating gases
Near drowning
Neoplasia*
Paraquat toxicity
Pneumonia/infectious disease*
- Aspiration/inhalation pneumonia
- Bacterial, e.g.
  - *Bordetella bronchiseptica*
  - *Chlamydophila psittaci*
  - *Escherichia coli*
  - *Klebsiella pneumoniae*
  - *Mycobacterium* spp.
  - *Mycoplasma pneumoniae*
  - Pasteurellosis
- Endogenous lipid pneumonia
- Fungal, e.g.
  - Aspergillosis
  - Blastomycosis
  - Coccidioidomycosis
  - Cryptococcosis
  - Histoplasmosis
  - Pneumocystis
- Parasitic, e.g.
  - *Aelurostrongylus abstrusus*
  - *Angiostrongylus vasorum*
  - *Capillaria aerophila*
  - *Crenosoma vulpis*
  - *Oslerus* spp.
  - *Paragonimus kellicotti*
  - Visceral larval migrans
- Protozoal, e.g.
  - Toxoplasmosis
- Rickettsial
- Viral, e.g.
  - Canine distemper virus* (D)
  - Feline calicivirus* (C)
  - Feline immunodeficiency virus* (C)
  - Feline leukaemia virus* (C)
Pulmonary oedema *q.v.*

Pulmonary thromboembolism, e.g.
- Cardiac disease
- Heartworm disease
- Hyperadrenocorticism

Smoke inhalation

Trauma, e.g.
- Pulmonary contusions
- Pulmonary haemorrhage

Restrictive disorders

Diaphragmatic hernia, e.g.
- Peritoneopericardial diaphragmatic hernia
- Traumatic*

Large intra-abdominal mass

Neoplasia
- Mediastinal
- Thoracic wall

Pickwickian syndrome (extreme obesity)

Pleural effusion* *q.v.*

Pneumothorax* *q.v.*

Severe ascites *q.v.*

Severe gastric distension

Severe hepatomegaly *q.v.*

Thoracic wall abnormalities, e.g.
- Neoplasia
- Pectus excavatum
- Trauma*

Systemic and miscellaneous disorders

Anaemia* *q.v.*

Central neurological disease causing damage to respiratory centres, e.g.
- Head trauma
- Hyperthermia* *q.v.*
- Hyperthyroidism* (C)
- Hypoxia*
- Metabolic acidosis *q.v.*
- Neuromuscular weakness, e.g. polyradiculoneuritis
- Shock/hypovolaemia* *q.v.*

Acute respiratory distress syndrome
Aspiration of acidic substances
Drug reaction
Inhalation injury
Lung lobe torsion
Multiple transfusions
Pancreatitis
Sepsis
Shock
Surgery
Trauma

2.3.2 Pallor

Anaemia q.v.

Decreased peripheral perfusion
Shock *q.v.*
Syncope
Vasoconstriction

Drugs/toxins
Adder bites
Baclofen
Diclofenac sodium
Ibuprofen
Ivermectin
Metaldehyde
Naproxen
Paracetamol
Vitamin D rodenticides

2.3.3 Shock

Cardiogenic

Decreased systolic function
Dilated cardiomyopathy*

Drugs/toxins, e.g.
- Doxorubicin

Myocardial infarction

Myocarditis

Decreased ventricular filling

Hypertrophic cardiomyopathy* (C)

Pericardial effusion/tamponade*

Restrictive cardiomyopathy* (C)

Restrictive pericarditis

Obstruction

Heartworm disease

Intracardiac mass

Thrombosis

Severe arrhythmia q.v.

Valve disease

Severe myxomatous degeneration of mitral valve* (D)

Rupture of chordae tendinae

Distributive

Anaphylactic

Septic

Hypovolaemic

Haemorrhage* *q.v.*

Hypoadrenocorticism (D)

Dehydration, e.g.

Diabetic ketoacidosis*

Diarrhoea* *q.v.*

Prolonged use of diuretics

Renal disease* *q.v.*

Vomiting* *q.v.*

Hypoproteinaemia/plasma loss, e.g.

Abdominal surgery

Ascites *q.v.*

Burns

Peripheral oedema *q.v.*

Pleural effusion

Hypoxaemic
Anaemia* *q.v.*
Respiratory disease* *q.v.*
Toxins
- Carbon monoxide
- Paracetamol

Metabolic
Heat stroke*
Hypoglycaemia
Sepsis*
Toxins, e.g.
- Cyanide

Neurogenic
Acute central nervous system disease
Electrocution
Heat stroke

2.3.4 Cyanosis

PERIPHERAL

Arterial obstruction, e.g.
Aortic thromboembolism* (C)

Vasoconstriction
Hypothermia* *q.v.*
Reduced cardiac output*
Shock* *q.v.*

Venous obstruction, e.g.
Right-sided heart failure*
Thrombophlebitis
Tourniquet

CENTRAL

Drugs/toxins
Baclofen
Blue-green algae

Loperamide
Metaldehyde
Paracetamol (and other causes of methaemoglobinaemia)
Paraquat
Theobromine

Hypoxaemia

Cardiovascular disease (anatomic shunts), e.g.
Pulmonary arteriovenous fistula
Reverse-shunting patent ductus arteriosus
Reverse-shunting ventricular septal defect
Tetralogy of Fallot

Haemoglobin abnormalities

Reduced inspired oxygen
Altitude
Anaesthetic

Respiratory disease
Hypoventilation
- Pleural effusion* *q.v.*
- Pneumothorax* *q.v.*
- Respiratory muscle failure
- Toxicity

Obstruction
- Brachycephalic obstructive airway syndrome
- Foreign body
  - Laryngeal
  - Tracheal
- Large mass in airway, e.g.
  - Abscess
  - Neoplasia
  - Parasite
- Laryngeal paralysis*

Ventilation–perfusion mismatch
- Acute respiratory distress syndrome
- Chronic obstructive pulmonary disease*
- Pneumonia
- Pulmonary inflammatory disease
- Pulmonary neoplasia*

- Pulmonary oedema* *q.v.*
- Pulmonary thromboembolism

2.3.5 Ascites (see Section 3.7.10 for full listing)

Bile
Blood
Chyle
Exudate
Transudate/modified transudate
Urine

2.3.6 Abnormal respiratory sounds

Crackles
Exudate in airways*
Haemorrhage in airways
Pulmonary fibrosis
Pulmonary oedema* *q.v.*

Stertor

Nasopharyngeal obstruction, e.g.
Brachycephalic obstructive airway syndrome
Foreign body*
Neoplasia

Stridor

Upper airway obstruction
Brachycephalic obstructive airway syndrome
Laryngeal obstruction, e.g.
- Foreign body
- Laryngospasm
- Neoplasia
- Oedema
- Paralysis*
Tracheal obstruction, e.g.
- Collapse*
- Extraluminal compression

- Exudate
- Foreign body
- Haemorrhage
- Neoplasia
- Stenosis

Wheezes

Airway narrowing, e.g.
Bronchoconstriction*
Extraluminal compression
Exudate in airways*
Masses in airways

2.3.7 Abnormal heart sounds

TRANSIENT HEART SOUNDS (HEART SOUNDS OF SHORT DURATION)

Loud S1

Anaemia* *q.v.*
Intensity varies with arrhythmias, e.g.
- Atrial fibrillation
- Heart block
- Sinus arrhythmia*
- Ventricular premature depolarisations*
High sympathetic tone*
Mitral insufficiency*
Systemic hypertension* *q.v.*
Tachycardia* *q.v.*
Thin animals*
Young animals*

Quiet S1

Decreased myocardial contractility, e.g.
- Dilated cardiomyopathy*
Diaphragmatic hernia*
Emphysema
First-degree heart block*

Obesity*
Pericardial effusion *q.v.*
Pleural effusion* *q.v.*
Shock* *q.v.*

Split S1
Bundle branch block
Cardiac pacing
Ectopic beats*
Physiological in healthy large-breed dogs*

Note: A split S1 should be differentiated from presystolic gallop, ejection sounds and diastolic clicks.

Loud S2
Anaemia* *q.v.*
Fever* *q.v.*
Hyperthyroidism* (C)
Intensity varies with arrhythmias, e.g.
- Atrial fibrillation
- Heart block
- Sinus arrhythmia*
- Ventricular premature depolarisations*
Tachycardia* *q.v.*
Thin animals*
Young animals*

Quiet S2
Decreased myocardial contractility, e.g.
- Dilated cardiomyopathy*
Diaphragmatic hernia*
Emphysema
Obesity*
Pericardial effusion *q.v.*
Pleural effusion* *q.v.*
Thoracic masses*
Shock* *q.v.*

Split S2
Physiological in healthy large-breed dogs*

Aortic valve closure follows pulmonic valve closure (A2 follows P2)
    Aortic stenosis
    Left bundle branch block
    Systemic hypertension
    Ventricular ectopic beats*

Pulmonic valve closure follows aortic valve closure (P2 follows A2)

Left to right intracardiac shunt (atrial septal defect)
    Pulmonary hypertension, e.g.
      • Heartworm disease
    Pulmonic stenosis
    Right bundle branch block
    Ventricular ectopic beats*

Gallop rhythms

Accentuated S3 (protodiastolic)
    Occasionally noted in healthy animals
    on phonocardiography
    Anaemia* *q.v.*
    Hyperthyroidism* (C)
    Mitral regurgitation*
    Myocardial dysfunction*
    Patent ductus arteriosus
    Septal defects

Accentuated S4 (presystolic)
    Inaudible in healthy animals, but may be noted
    on phonocardiography
    Hyperthyroidism* (C)
    Hypertrophic cardiomyopathy* (C)
    Marked left ventricular hypertrophy
    Profound heart failure following rupture of chordae tendinae

Early diastolic sounds

    Opening snaps (rare)
      • Mitral valve stenosis
    Pericardial knocks
      • Constrictive pericarditis
    Plops
      • Mobile atrial tumours

Ejection sounds (high frequency sounds in early diastole)
    Aortic stenosis
    Dilatation of the great vessels
    Heartworm disease
    Hypertension* *q.v.*
    Opening of abnormal semilunar valves
    Pulmonic stenosis
    Tetralogy of Fallot

Systolic clicks (short, mid- to high-frequency sounds in mid to late systole)
    Early degenerative valvular disease

MURMURS (HEART SOUNDS OF LONGER DURATION ARISING FROM TURBULENT BLOOD FLOW)

Innocent murmurs*

Physiological murmurs
    Anaemia* *q.v.*
    Fever* *q.v.*
    Hypertension* *q.v.*
    Hyperthyroidism* (C)
    Pregnancy*

Murmurs associated with cardiovascular disease

Continuous
    Coronary arteriovenous fistula
    Coronary artery or ruptured sinus aneurysm communicating directly with right atrium
    Patent ductus arteriosus
    Pulmonary arteriovenous fistula

Diastolic
    Aortic insufficiency (congenital or associated with bacterial endocarditis)
    Mitral stenosis

Systolic
    Holosystolic crescendo–decrescendo
    • Aortic stenosis
    • Pulmonic stenosis
    • Ventricular septal defect

Holosystolic plateau-shaped
- Mitral regurgitation*
- Tricuspid regurgitation*
- Ventricular septal defect

2.3.8   Abnormalities in heart rate

BRADYCARDIA
Normal in athletic dogs, during rest/sleep
Cardiac disease/arrhythmias *q.v.*
CNS disease
Hypothermia
Severe systemic disease

Drugs/toxins
Adder bites
Amiodarone
Antidysrhythmics, e.g. beta blockers
Atenolol
Baclofen
Bethanechol
Cannabis
Carbamate
Clonidine
Daffodil
Diltiazem
Fentanyl
Glyphosate
Hypertonic saline
Ivermectin
Lignocaine
Loperamide
Medetomidine
Mexiletine
Organophosphates
Paraquat
Phenoxy acid herbicides
Propranolol
Pyridostigmine

Rhododendron
Sotalol
Theobromine
Timolol maleate
Verapamil
Vitamin D rodenticides
Xylazine
Yew

Increased vagal tone*, e.g.
Gastrointestinal disease* *q.v.*
Respiratory disease* *q.v.*

Metabolic disease
Hyperkalaemia *q.v.*
Hypoadrenocorticism
Hypoglycaemia *q.v.*
Hypothyroidism*
Uraemia*

TACHYCARDIA

Drugs/toxins
Adder bites
Adrenaline
Atropine
Baclofen
Blue-green algae
Cannabis
Dinoprost tromethamine
Dobutamine
Dopamine
Doxapram
Doxorubicin
Ethylene glycol
Glyceryl trinitrate
Glycopyrronium bromide
Glyphosate
Hydralazine
Ibuprofen
Isosorbide dinitrate

Ketamine
Levothyroxine
Metaldehyde
Paracetamol
Paraquat
Petroleum distillates
Phenoxy acid herbicides
Phenoxybenzamine
Propantheline bromide
Pyrethrins/pyrethroids
Salbutamol
Selective serotonin reuptake inhibitors
Terbutaline
Terfenadine
Theobromine
Theophylline
Tricyclic antidepressants
Verapamil
Vitamin D rodenticides

Sinus tachycardia

Physiological
  Excitement*
  Exercise*
  Fear*
  Pain*

Pathological
  Heart failure*
  Respiratory disease*
  Shock*
  Systemic disease
    • Anaemia* *q.v.*
    • Fever* *q.v.*
    • Hyperthyroidism (C)*
    • Hypoxia*
    • Sepsis*

Other types of supraventricular tachycardia* q.v.

Ventricular tachycardia* q.v.

2.3.9 Jugular distension/hepatojugular reflux

Cardiac disease resulting in right-sided heart failure*
Fluid volume overload, e.g.
* Iatrogenic*
Pericardial disease

2.3.10 Alterations in arterial pulse

Hyperkinetic (bounding) pulse
Anaemia* *q.v.*
Arteriovenous fistula
Bradycardia* *q.v.*
Decreased diastolic blood pressure
* Aortic insufficiency
* Shunting lesions, e.g.
  - Increased stroke volume
  - Increased systolic blood pressure
  - Patent ductus arteriosus
Fever* *q.v.*
Hyperthyroidism* (c)

Hypokinetic (weak) pulse
Aortic stenosis
Increased peripheral resistance
Regional loss of pulse (see succeeding text
Small stroke volume, e.g.
* Hypovolaemia* *q.v.*
* Left-sided heart failure*
Tachycardia *q.v.*
Toxins
* Alphachloralose
* Anticoagulant rodenticides

Pulsus alternans
Myocardial failure
Tachyarrhythmias *q.v.*

Pulsus bigeminus
Ventricular bigeminy

Pulse deficits
Tachyarrhythmias *q.v.*

Pulsus paradoxus
Exaggerated in pericardial effusion (with cardiac tamponade)
Physiological

Regional loss of pulse
Infectious embolus
Neoplastic embolus
Thromboembolism*

2.4 Dermatological signs

2.4.1 Scaling

Exfoliative dermatoses
Contact dermatitis*
Drug eruption
Epitheliotrophic lymphoma
Feline immunodeficiency virus* (C)
Feline leukaemia virus* (C)
Parapsoriasis
Pemphigus foliaceus
Systemic lupus erythematosus
Thymoma
Toxic epidermal necrolysis

Primary/inherited disorders of keratinisation
Acne*
Canine primary idiopathic seborrhoea (D)
Ear margin dermatosis
Epidermal dysplasia (Armadillo Westie syndrome) (D)
Feline idiopathic facial dermatitis (C)
Feline primary idiopathic seborrhoea (C)

Follicular dysplasia
Follicular hyperkeratosis
Follicular parakeratosis
Footpad hyperkeratosis
Ichthyosis
Lethal acrodermatitis
Lichenoid psoriasiform dermatosis
Nasal hyperkeratosis*
Nasodigital hyperkeratosis
Schnauzer comedo syndrome (D)
Sebaceous adenitis
Tail gland hyperplasia*
Vitamin-A-responsive dermatosis
Zinc-responsive dermatosis

Secondary scaling

Allergic/immune-mediated
Atopy*
Contact hypersensitivity
Drug hypersensitivity
Food hypersensitivity*
Hormonal hypersensitivity
Pemphigus foliaceus

Environmental
Low humidity
Physical/chemical damage

Infectious/parasitic
Bacterial pyoderma
Cheyletiellosis*
Cowpox virus (C)
Demodecosis*
Dermatophytosis*
Endoparasites*
Fleas*
Leishmaniasis
Malassezia spp*
Pediculosis*
Pyoderma*
Scabies* (D)

Metabolic/endocrine
　　Diabetic dermatopathy
　　Growth hormone-responsive dermatosis
　　Hepatic disease
　　Hyperadrenocorticism
　　Hyperandrogenism
　　Hyperthyroidism* (C)
　　Hypopituitarism
　　Hypothyroidism* (D)
　　Idiopathic male feminising syndrome
　　Intestinal disease
　　Necrolytic migratory erythema
　　Oestrogen-responsive dermatosis
　　Pancreatic disease
　　Renal disease
　　Sertoli cell tumour
　　Sex hormone abnormalities
　　Superficial necrolytic dermatitis
　　　　• Glucagonoma
　　　　• Hepatocutaneous syndrome
　　Testosterone-responsive dermatosis

Neoplastic
　　Epitheliotrophic lymphoma

Nutritional
　　Dietary deficiency of essential fatty acids
　　Malabsorption/malnutrition of essential fatty acids

2.4.2 Pustules and papules (including miliary dermatitis)

Primary immune-mediated
　　Bullous pemphigoid
　　Pemphigus erythematosus
　　Pemphigus foliaceus
　　Pemphigus vegetans
　　Pemphigus vulgaris
　　Systemic lupus erythematosus

Immune-mediated diseases causing secondary pyoderma

Atopy*
Contact allergy*
Food hypersensitivity*
Hypereosinophilic syndrome

Infectious/parasitic diseases causing secondary pyoderma

Cheyletiellosis
Demodecosis*
Dermatophilosis
Dermatophytosis*
External parasite bites*, e.g.
- Fleas
- Mosquitoes

Feline immunodeficiency virus*
Feline leukaemia virus*
Lynxacarus radovskyi
Malassezia spp.*
Notoedres cati
Pediculosis*
Sarcoptic mange*
Superficial pustular dermatitis*
Trombiculiasis*

Miscellaneous

Canine linear IgA pustular dermatosis (D)
Contact irritation*
Drug eruptions
Juvenile cellulitis
Sterile eosinophilic pustular dermatosis
Subcorneal pustular dermatosis

Neoplastic

Epitheliotrophic lymphoma
Mast cell tumour*

Nutritional

Biotin deficiency
Essential fatty acid deficiency

2.4.3 Nodules

Inflammation

Angiogenic oedema
Calcinosis circumscripta
Calcinosis cutis
Infectious
- Bacterial*
- Fungal
- Parasitic

Granuloma, e.g.
- Eosinophilic*
- Insect bite*

Histiocytosis
Nodular cutaneous
amyloidosis
Nodular dermatofibrosis
Panniculitis
Sterile nodular granuloma
Urticaria*
Xanthoma

Neoplasia

Epithelial

Apocrine adenoma/carcinoma*
Basal cell tumour*
Ceruminous adenoma/carcinoma*
Keratoacanthoma*
Papilloma*
Perianal gland adenoma/carcinoma*
Pilomatrixoma*
Sebaceous adenoma/carcinoma*
Squamous cell carcinoma*
Sweat gland tumours*
Trichoepithelioma*

Melanocyte

Melanoma

Round cell
   Lymphoma
      • Epitheliotrophic
      • Lymphomatoid granulomatosis
      • Non-epitheliotrophic
   Histiocytic sarcoma
   Histiocytoma*
   Mast cell tumour*
   Plasmacytoma*
   Transmissible venereal tumour

Mesenchymal
   Benign fibrous histiocytoma
   Dermatofibroma
   Fibrolipoma
   Fibroma
   Fibropapilloma
   Fibrosarcoma
   Haemangioma/sarcoma
   Haemangiopericytoma
   Leiomyoma/sarcoma
   Lipoma/sarcoma*
   Lymphangioma/sarcoma
   Myxosarcoma
   Schwannoma

Metastatic

Non-neoplastic, non-inflammatory
   Benign nodular sebaceous hyperplasia
   Cysts*
      • Dermoid
      • Epidermoid
      • Follicular
   Fibroadnexal dysplasia
   Haematoma*
   Naevi/hamartoma
      • Collagenous
      • Follicular
      • Sebaceous
      • Vascular

Seroma*
Skin polyp*
Urticaria pigmentosa

2.4.4   Pigmentation disorders (coat or skin)

HYPOPIGMENTATION
Generalised
Age-related greying*
Albinism
Canine cyclic haematopoiesis (D)
Chediak–Higashi syndrome (C)
Mucocutaneous hypopigmentation
Nutritional deficiencies
  * Copper
  * Lysine
  * Pantothenic acid
  * Protein
  * Pyridoxine
  * Zinc
Oculocutaneous albinism
Piebaldism
Tyrosinase deficiency
Waardenburg syndrome
Drugs

Localised

Idiopathic
Periocular leukotrichia/Aguirre syndrome
Seasonal nasal hypopigmentation*

Immune-mediated
Sutton's halo
Uveodermatological syndrome
Vitiligo

Infectious
Aspergillosis
Leishmaniasis

Neoplastic
  Basal cell tumour
  Epitheliotrophic lymphoma
  Gastric carcinoma
  Mammary adenocarcinoma*
  Melanoma
  Squamous cell carcinoma

Post-inflammatory
  Bullous pemphigoid
  Inflammatory dermatitis* *q.v.*
  Lupus erythematosus

Trauma
  Burns
  Chemical
  Physical*
  Radiation
  Surgical*

HYPERPIGMENTATION

Drugs
  • Minocycline
  • Mitotane

Focal
  Acanthosis nigrans
  Demodecosis*
  Dermatophytosis*
  Lentigo
  Naevus
  Neoplasia*
  Post-inflammatory
  Pyoderma*
  Trauma*

Generalised/diffuse
  Alopecia X
  Demodecosis*
  Endocrine disease
    • Adrenal sex-hormone dermatosis

- Growth hormone-responsive dermatosis
- Hyperadrenocorticism
- Hyperoestrogenism
- Hypothyroidism* (D)

Iatrogenic

- Prolonged glucocorticoid administration

Malassezia spp.*

Recurrent flank alopecia

Ultraviolet irradiation of alopecic regions

Multifocal

Bowen's disease (C)

Demodecosis*

Dermatophytosis*

Lentigines

Melanoderma

Naevus

Post-inflammatory

Pyoderma*

Tumours*

Urticaria pigmentosa

2.4.5 Alopecia

Failure of hair growth

Paraneoplastic alopecia

Endocrine disease

Diabetes mellitus*

Hyperadrenocorticism

Hypothyroidism* (D)

Follicular diseases

Anagen defluvium

- Cancer chemotherapy
- Endocrine disease*
- Infection
- Metabolic disease*

Colour-dilution alopecia

Congenital follicular dysplasias

Congenital hypotrichosis
Dark hair follicular dystrophy

Hair cycle arrest alopecia
Endocrine disease
- Alopecia X
  - Adrenal sex hormone-responsive dermatosis
  - Castration-responsive dermatosis
  - Growth hormone-responsive dermatosis
  - Oestrogen responsive dermatosis
- Testosterone-responsive dermatosis
  - Hyperadrenocorticism
  - Hyperoestrogenism
  - Hypothyroidism* (D)
Idiopathic cyclic flank alopecia
Pattern baldness
Post-clipping
Telogen defluvium*
- Stress, e.g.
  - Anaesthesia
  - Pregnancy
  - Shock *q.v.*
  - Surgery
  - Systemic illness

Systemic diseases
Chronic hepatic disease *q.v.*
End-stage renal disease *q.v.*
Feline immunodeficiency virus (C)
Feline leukaemia virus (C)

Damage to hair follicle
Secondary to pruritus* *q.v.*

Drugs
- Carbimazole

Follicular infections
Bacterial folliculitis*
Demodecosis*
Dermatophytosis*

Immune-mediated disease
Alopecia areata
Idiopathic lymphocytic mural folliculitis
Pseudopelade
Sebaceous adenitis

Miscellaneous
Alopecia mucinosis
Feline-acquired symmetric alopecia (C)
Feline pinnal alopecia* (C)
Feline pre-auricular alopecia (normal)
Follicular lipidosis of Rottweilers (D)
Medullary trichomalacia
Psychogenic alopecia*
Short hair syndrome of Silky breeds (D)

*Neoplasia**

Nutritional
Zinc deficiency
Zinc-responsive dermatosis

Trauma/physical
Injection site reaction
Over-grooming
Sensory neuropathy
Traction alopecia
Trichoptilosis
Tricorrhexis nodosa

2.4.6   Erosive/ulcerative skin disease

Drugs/toxins
ACE inhibitors
Diuretics
Fenbendazole
Imodium
Itraconazole
Ivermectin
Metoclopramide

Metronidazole
Phenobarbitone
Phenylbutazone
Thallium

Idiopathic
Feline idiopathic ulcerative dermatosis

Immune-mediated
Bullous pemphigoid
Discoid lupus erythematosus
Epidermolysis bullosa acquisita
Erythema multiforme
Mucous membrane pemphigoid
Perianal fistulae
Plasma cell pododermatitis
Systemic lupus erythematosus
Toxic epidermal necrolysis
Ulcerative disease of Shetland Sheepdog
and Rough Collie (D)

Infection
Antibiotic responsive ulcerative
dermatoses
Cowpox virus (C)

Neoplasia*

Physical
Burns
Frostbite
Radiation
Trauma

Vasculitis
Idiopathic
Immune-mediated
Infectious

2.4.7   Otitis externa

Primary causes

Disorders of keratinisation
    Primary seborrhoea
    Sebaceous adenitis
    Vitamin-A-responsive dermatosis

Endocrine, e.g.
    Hyperadrenocorticism
    Hypothyroidism* (D)

Hypersensitivity
    Atopy*
    Contact allergy*
    Drug reactions
    Food hypersensitivity*

Immune-mediated
    Bullous pemphigoid
    Cold agglutinin disease
    Drug eruption
    Erythema multiforme
    Lupus erythematosus
    Pemphigus erythematosus
    Pemphigus foliaceus
    Vasculitis

Infection
    Fungal
- Dermatophytosis*
- *Sporothrix schenckii*

    Parasites
- Demodecosis*
- Fleas*
- *Otodectes cyanotis* *
- Pediculosis*
- Sarcoptic mange* (D)
- Trombiculosis*

    Pyoderma

Miscellaneous
  Abnormal cerumen production
  Juvenile cellulitis

Neoplasia
  Adenocarcinoma
  Adenoma
  Papilloma
  Squamous cell carcinoma

Physical
  Foreign body*

Predisposing factors

Ear conformation/structure
  Ear canal stenosis
    • Acquired*
    • Inherited
  Hypertrichosis*
  Neoplasia
  Pendulous pinnae* (D)
  Polyps*

Excessive moisture
  Humidity
  Swimming

Iatrogenic

Irritant ear cleaning products
  Overuse of cleaning products
  Trauma

Systemic immunosuppression

Perpetuating factors
  Acquired changes secondary to chronic ear disease
    • Fibrosis*
    • Hyperplasia*
    • Mineralisation*
    • Oedema*
    • Ulceration*

Bacterial infection*
- *Enterobacter* spp.
- *Proteus* spp.
- *Pseudomonas* spp
- *Staphylococcus intermedius*
- *Streptococcus* spp.

Candidiasis*

Otitis media

2.4.8 Pododermatitis

Asymmetric pododermatitis

Infection

Bacterial*
- *Actinomyces* spp.
- *Nocardia* spp.
- *Proteus* spp.
- *Pseudomonas* spp
- *Staphylococcus intermedius*

Fungal
- Blastomycosis
- Candidiasis
- Cryptococcosis
- Dermatophytosis*
- Eumycotic mycetoma
- *Malassezia** spp.

Parasitic, e.g.
- Demodecosis*

Miscellaneous

Acral lick dermatitis*

Arteriovenous fistula

Calcinosis circumscripta

Foreign body*

Irritant*

Osteomyelitis

Sensory neuropathy

Neoplasia

Trauma

Symmetric pododermatitis

Congenital
    Acrodermatitis of Bull Terriers (D)
    Familial hyperkeratosis in Irish Terriers (D)
    Familial vasculopathy of German Shepherd (D)
    Idiopathic footpad hyperkeratosis
    Tyrosinaemia
    Vasculitis of Jack Russell Terriers (D)

Immunodeficiencies
    Acquired
    Congenital

Immune-mediated/allergic
    Atopy*
    Bullous pemphigoid
    Cold agglutinins
    Contact allergy*
    Dermatomyositis (D)
    Drug eruption
    Food allergy*
    Pemphigus foliaceus
    Pemphigus vulgaris
    Plasma cell pododermatitis (C)
    Sterile granuloma/pyogranuloma
    Systemic lupus erythematosus
    Vasculitis

Infection
    Bacterial, e.g.
      • *Staphylococcus intermedius*
    Fungal, e.g.
      • *Malassezia* spp.
    Parasitic, e.g.
      • Demodecosis
      • Hookworm
      • Leishmaniasis
      • *Pelodera*
    Viral
      • Distemper* (D)

Irritant

Metabolic
   Calcinosis circumscripta
   Superficial necrolytic dermatitis

Miscellaneous
   Dermatofibrosis

Neoplasia

Nutritional
   Zinc responsive dermatosis

Psychogenic/neurogenic
   Acral mutilation of German
   Short-Haired Pointers (D)
   Sensory neuropathy

2.4.9   Disorders of the claws

Drugs/toxins
   Thallotoxicosis

Idiopathic conditions
   Idiopathic onychodystrophy
   Idiopathic onychogryphosis
   Idiopathic onychomadesis

Immune-mediated disease
   Bullous pemphigoid
   Cryoglobulinaemia
   Discoid lupus erythematosus/symmetric
   lupoid onychodystrophy
   Drug eruption
   Eosinophilic granuloma complex
   Pemphigus complex
   Systemic lupus erythematosus
   Vasculitis

Infection
　Bacterial
　　• Secondary to trauma or virus*
　Fungal
　　• Blastomycosis
　　• Candidiasis
　　• Cryptococcosis
　　• Dermatophytosis
　　• Geotrichosis
　　• *Malassezia* spp.
　　• Sporothricosis
　Parasitic
　　• Ascarids
　　• Demodecosis
　　• Hookworm dermatitis
　Protozoal
　　• Leishmaniasis
　Viral
　　• Canine distemper virus* (D)
　　• Feline immunodeficiency virus* (C)
　　• Feline leukaemia virus* (C)

Inherited/primary disease
　Anonychia (loss of nails)
　Dermatomyositis
　Epidermolysis bullosa
　Naevus
　Primary seborrhoea
　Supernumerary claws

Metabolic/endocrine disease
　Acromegaly
　Diabetes mellitus*
　Hyperadrenocorticism
　Hyperthyroidism* (C)
　Hypothyroidism* (D)
　Necrolytic migratory erythema

Neoplasia, e.g.
　Metastatic lung carcinoma
　Squamous cell carcinoma

Nutrition

Lethal acrodermatitis
Zinc responsive dermatosis

Trauma

Irritant chemical*
Physical injury*

Vascular

Disseminated intravascular coagulation
Raynaud-like disease

2.4.10   Anal sac/perianal disease

Perianal/caudal pruritus

Anal sac impaction*
Anal sacculitis*
Atopy*
Flea bite hypersensitivity*
Food hypersensitivity*
Intertrigo*
- Perineal
- Tail fold
- Vulval fold
Parasitism*, e.g.
- Cheyletiellosis
- Sarcoptic mange

Perianal fistula

Anal furunculosis*
Ruptured anal sac abscess*

Perianal swelling

Anal sac abscess*
Anal sac neoplasia*
Perianal adenoma*
Other perianal neoplasia
Perineal hernia*
Rectal prolapse*

2.5 Neurological signs

2.5.1 Abnormal cranial nerve (CN) responses

The anatomical localisation of lesions associated with the abnormal test are listed, together with other disorders that can produce alterations in the cranial nerve tests.

Anisocoria

Abnormal pupil constricted
  Corneal ulcers/lacerations
  Drugs, e.g.
  • Pilocarpine
  Horner syndrome
  Posterior synechiae
  Previous inflammation
  Uveitis*

Abnormal pupil dilated
  Iris, retina, CN II, CN III
  • Chorioretinitis
  • Glaucoma
  • Iris atrophy/hypoplasia
  • Iris trauma
  • Posterior synechiae
  • Unilateral blindness
  • Drugs, e.g.
    ○ Atropine
    ○ Phenylephrine

Auditory response reduced
  CN VIII
  External auditory canal*
  Middle* or inner ear

Corneal reflex reduced
  Brainstem
  CN V
  CN VII

Facial asymmetry

Facial paralysis
- CN VII
- Idiopathic neuritis
- Neoplasia of the middle ear
- Otitis media*

Masticatory muscle wastage
- CN V
  - Idiopathic trigeminal neuritis
  - Malignant trigeminal nerve sheath tumour
- Masticatory myositis

Gag reflex reduced

Brainstem
CN IX
CN X

Jaw tone reduced/inability to close jaw

CN V
- Idiopathic trigeminal neuritis
- Lymphoma*
- Neosporosis

Orthopaedic or muscular disease

Lack of response to non-irritant smell

CN I
Nasal disease

Menace response reduced

Brainstem
Cerebellum
CN II
CN VII
Forebrain
Immature animal
Retina

Palpebral reflex reduced

Brainstem
CN V
CN VII

Pupillary light reflex reduced
Brainstem
CN II
CN III
Retina

Response to stimulation of nasal mucosa reduced
Brainstem
CN V
Forebrain

Response to vagal manoeuvres reduced
CN X

Spontaneous nystagmus
Brainstem
CN VIII
Toxic, e.g.
- Cannabis
- Metaldehyde

Vestibular disease *q.v.*, e.g.
- Canine idiopathic geriatric vestibular disease*
- Congenital vestibular disease
- Middle ear disease

Strabismus

Ventrolateral
CN III

Dorsolateral
CN IV

Medial
CN VI

Vestibulo-ocular reflex reduced
Brainstem
CN III
CN IV
CN VI
CN VIII

Diseases of CN V
Idiopathic trigeminal neuritis
Infiltrating neoplasia, e.g.
- Lymphoma
- Nerve sheath tumours

Diseases of CN VII
Idiopathic
Insulinoma
Otitis media/interna
Trauma of middle ear
Tumour of middle ear

2.5.2 Vestibular disease

(Signs include head tilt, nystagmus, circling, leaning, falling and rolling)

PERIPHERAL VESTIBULAR SYSTEM
Congenital vestibular disease
Drugs/toxins

Antibiotics
Aminoglycosides
Amphotericin B
Ampicillin
Bacitracin
Chloramphenicol
Colistin
Erythromycin
Griseofulvin
Hygromycin B
Metronidazole
Minocycline
Polymixin B
Tetracyclines
Vancomycin

Antiseptics
Benzalkonium chloride
Benzethonium chloride

Cetrimide
Chlorhexidine
Ethanol
Iodine
Iodophores

Cancer chemotherapeutics
Actinomycin
Cisplatin
Cyclophosphamide
Vinblastine
Vincristine

Diuretics
Bumetanide
Ethacrynic acid
Frusemide

Metals/heavy metals
Arsenic
Gold salts
Lead
Mercury
Triethyl/trimethyl tin

Miscellaneous
Ceruminolytic agents
Danazol
Detergents
Digoxin
Dimethylsulphoxide
Diphenylhydrazine
Insulin
Mexiletine
Potassium bromide
Prednisolone
Propylene glycol
Quinidine
Salicylates

Idiopathic conditions
Idiopathic geriatric vestibular disease*

Infection
Extension of otitis externa* *q.v.*
Foreign bodies*
Haematogenous spread of infection
Otitis media/interna*
Polyps*

Metabolic disease
Hypothyroidism* (D)

Neoplasia
Ceruminous gland adenocarcinoma
Chondrosarcoma
Fibrosarcoma
Osteosarcoma
Schwannoma
Squamous cell carcinoma

Trauma

CENTRAL VESTIBULAR SYSTEM
Congenital conditions
Chiari-like malformation
Hydrocephalus

Degeneration
Lysosomal storage disorders

Drugs/toxins
Metronidazole

Idiopathic conditions
Arachnoid cysts

Immune-mediated/Infection
Feline spongiform encephalopathy (C)
Meningoencephalitis

Metabolic disease
Electrolyte abnormalities* *q.v.*
Hepatic encephalopathy* *q.v.*
Uraemic encephalopathy* *q.v.*

Neoplasia
Choroid plexus tumours
Dermoid cyst
Epidermoid cyst
Glioma
Lymphoma
Medulloblastoma
Meningioma
Metastatic tumour

Nutrition
Thiamine deficiency
Trauma

Vascular disorders
Cerebrovascular accident

2.5.3   Horner's syndrome

First order (hypothalamus, rostral midbrain, spinal cord to T3)
Intracranial disease, e.g.
- Neoplasia

Spinal disease *q.v.*
Thoracic disease, e.g.
- Cranial mediastinal mass

Second order (pre-ganglionic) (T1–T3, vagosympathetic trunk, caudal and cranial cervical ganglia)
Brachial plexus avulsion
Cervical soft tissue disease, e.g.
- Mass
- Neoplasia
- Trauma

Cervical surgery, e.g.
- Thyroidectomy

Third order (post-ganglionic) (middle ear, cranial cavity, eye)
Feline immunodeficiency virus* (C)

Iatrogenic, e.g.
- Bulla osteotomy

Idiopathic*

Middle ear
- Mass
- Neoplasia

Otitis media/interna*

Retrobulbar
- Injury
- Mass*
- Neoplasia

2.5.4 Hemineglect syndrome (Forebrain dysfunction q.v.)

2.5.5 Spinal disorders

C1–C5

Acute

Atlantoaxial subluxation
Cervical spondylomyelopathy (D)
Degenerative disc disease* (D)
Discospondylitis
Fibrocartilaginous embolism*
Fracture*
Granulomatous meningoencephalomyelitis
Haematoma
Ischaemic myelopathy
Luxation
Neoplasia

Chronic

Atlanto-occipital dysplasia
Atlantoaxial subluxation
Calcinosis circumscripta
Cervical fibrotic stenosis
Cervical spondylomyelopathy* (D)
Feline infectious peritonitis (C)

Hypervitaminosis A
Neoplasia
Spinal arachnoid cysts
Synovial cysts
Syringohydromyelia*

C6–T2

Acute

Brachial plexus avulsion
Cervical spondylomyelopathy* (D)
Degenerative disc disease* (D)
Discospondylitis
Fibrocartilaginous embolism*
Fracture*
Granulomatous meningoencephalomyelitis
Haematoma
Luxation
Neoplasia

Chronic

Cervical spondylomyelopathy* (D)
Dermoid sinus
Neoplasia
Spinal arachnoid cysts
Synovial cysts

T3–L3

Acute

Ascending myelomalacia
Degenerative disc disease* (D)
Discospondylitis
Fibrocartilaginous embolism
Fracture*
Granulomatous meningoencephalomyelitis
Luxation
Neoplasia

Chronic

Calcinosis circumscripta
Degenerative disc disease* (D)

Degenerative myelopathy*
Neoplasia
Spinal arachnoid cyst
Synovial cysts

L4–S3

Acute
Ascending myelomalacia
Cauda equina neuritis* (D)
Degenerative disc disease* (D)
Discospondylitis
Fibrocartilaginous embolism
Fracture*
Granulomatous meningoencephalomyelitis
Ischaemic neuromyopathy
Luxation
Neoplasia
Psoas muscle injury

Chronic
Degenerative myelopathy*
Dermoid sinus
Lumbosacral disc disease* (D)
Neoplasia
Sacral osteochondritis dissecans
Sacrocaudal dysgenesis
Spina bifida
Tethered cord syndrome

2.6   Ocular signs

2.6.1   Red eye

CONJUNCTIVITIS
Chemical
Acid
Alkali

Antiseptics
Shampoos

Immune-mediated
Allergic
Arthropod bites*
Atopy*
Drug reaction
Food hypersensitivity*
Idiopathic
Keratoconjunctivitis sicca*

Infectious
Bacterial*
Fungal, e.g.
  • Blastomycosis
Mycoplasmal
Parasitic, e.g.
  • Thelazia spp.
Rickettsial
Viral, e.g.
  • Canine distemper virus* (D)

Neurological
Lack of blink reflex
  • Lesions of facial nerve *q.v.*
  • Lesions of trigeminal nerve *q.v.*
Lack of tear production
  • Neurogenic keratoconjunctivitis sicca

Physical
Cilia*
Dust*
Foreign body*
Masses*
Poor eyelid anatomy*
  • Ectropion
  • Entropion
Radiation therapy

Neoplastic, e.g.

Mast cell tumour
Melanoma
Squamous cell carcinoma

Systemic diseases

Hepatozoonosis
Leishmaniasis
Listeriosis
Multiple myeloma
Systemic histiocytosis
Tyrosinaemia (D)

ANTERIOR UVEITIS

Idiopathic

Ionising radiation

Infection

Algae

Prototothecosis

Bacteria

Bartonella
Borreliosis
Brucellosis (D)
Leptospirosis
Septicaemia
- Abscesses*
- Bacterial endocarditis
- Dental infections*
- Neonatal umbilical infections
- Prostatitis*
- Pyelonephritis
- Pyometra*
- Pyothorax

Fungal

Blastomycosis
Candidiasis

   Coccidioidomycosis
   Cryptococcosis
   Histoplasmosis

Parasitic
   Angiostrongylosis
   Baylisascaris procyonis
   Diptera
   Dirofilariasis
   Toxocariasis

Protozoa
   Leishmaniasis
   Neosporosis (D)
   Toxoplasmosis

Rickettsia
   Ehrlichiosis
   Rocky Mountain Spotted Fever

Viruses
   Canine adenovirus-1 (D)
   Canine distemper virus
   Canine herpes virus (D)
   Feline immunodeficiency virus (C)*
   Feline infectious peritonitis (C)*
   Feline leukaemia virus (C)*
   Rabies

Neoplasia
   Adenocarcinomas
   Ciliary body
   Ciliary body adenoma
   Medulloepitheliomas
   Melanoma
   Metastatic neoplasia, especially
     • Haemangiosarcoma
     • Lymphoma
   Sarcoma
   Systemic histiocytosis

Non-infectious inflammatory

Lens-associated anterior uveitis
- Cataract*
- Luxation*
- Penetrating trauma*

Granulomatous meningoencephalomyelitis
Idiopathic
Immune-mediated vasculitis
Pigmentary uveitis
Uveodermatological syndrome

Systemic, e.g.

Coagulopathy
Hyperlipidaemia *q.v.*
Systemic hypertension* *q.v.*
Toxaemia

Trauma

Blunt trauma*
Penetrating trauma*/intraocular
foreign bodies
Drugs, e.g.
- Miotics

BULBAR HYPERAEMIA/VASCULAR CONGESTION

Anterior scleritis
Trauma*

Episcleritis

Nodular
Simple

Glaucoma

Primary

Goniodysgenesis
Primary open angle glaucoma

Secondary

Cataract* *q.v.*

Drugs
- Atropine
- Sildenafil

Intraocular haemorrhage* *q.v.*
Lens luxation*
Neoplasia
Neovascular tissue overlying pectinate ligament
Pigmentary glaucoma
Trauma
Uveitis* *q.v.*
Vitreous prolapse post-lentectomy

Cornea Red

Haemorrhage
Granulation tissue
Neovascularisation

Intraocular Red Eye

Anterior uveitis
Hyphaema
Iris mass
Retinal detachment
Vitreal haemorrhage

2.6.2   Corneal opacification

Corneal oedema

Anterior uveitis* *q.v.*
Canine adenovirus-1 (D)
Corneal ulceration* *q.v.*
Drugs/toxins
- Tocainide

Endophthalmitis
Endothelial dystrophy
Glaucoma *q.v.*
Historic use of canine adenovirus-1 live vaccine
Intraocular neoplasia
Mechanical trauma*/iatrogenic

Neovascularisation
Persistent pupillary membranes

Corneal vascularisation

Endophthalmitis
Glaucoma *q.v.*
Intraocular neoplasia
Keratitis*
Pannus*
Uveitis* *q.v.*

Miscellaneous

Calcium deposition
Cellular infiltration
Degenerative changes
Foreign bodies*
Lipid deposition
Neoplastic infiltration
Scarring*
Xerosis

Pigmentation

Anterior synechiae
Chronic corneal insult*
Congenital endothelial pigmentation
Corneal sequestrum
Limbal melanoma
Persistent pupillary membranes
Pigmentary glaucoma

2.6.3   Corneal ulceration/erosion

Degeneration

Corneal calcific degeneration
Lipid keratopathy

Dystrophic

Bullous keratopathy
Corneal endothelial dystrophy

Corneal sequestrum (C)
Epithelial basement membrane dystrophy (indolent ulcer)

Infection

Bacterial (secondary invaders)
   Bacillus spp.
   Corynebacterium spp.
   Escherichia coli
   Pseudomonas spp.
   Staphylococcus spp.
   Streptococcus spp.

Fungal
   Acremonium spp.
   Alternaria spp.
   Aspergillosis
   Candidiasis
   Cephalosporium spp.
   Curvalia spp.
   Pseudallescheria spp.
   Scedosporium spp.

Protozoal

Viral
   Feline herpes virus* (C)

Inflammation/immune-mediated

   Feline eosinophilic keratitis
   Keratoconjunctivitis sicca*
   Punctate keratopathy (D)

Mechanical/irritant trauma

   Aberrant hairs*
   Distichiasis*
   Ectopic cilia*
   Eyelid abnormalities*
      • Ectropion
      • Entropion
   Heat
   Irritant chemicals

Self-trauma*
Shampoos
Smoke*
Trichiasis*
Ultraviolet light*

Neurological conditions
Ionising radiation
Lack of blink reflex
- Lesions of facial nerve *q.v.*
- Lesions of trigeminal nerve *q.v.*
Lack of tear production
- Neurogenic keratoconjunctivitis sicca

2.6.4   Lens lesions

Cataract
Age-related*
Electrocution
Glaucoma *q.v.*
Lens luxation (see succeeding text)
Non-hereditary developmental
Post-inflammation
Radiation
Retinal degeneration

Drugs/toxins
Diazoxide
Dimethyl sulfoxide
Dinitrophenol
Hydroxymethylglutaryl-coenzyme A reductase inhibitors
Ketoconazole
Pefloxacin
Phenylpiperazine
Progesterone-based contraceptives
Sulfonylurea glimepiride
Topical dexamethasone

Hereditary, e.g.
Congenital with microphthalmos and rotatory nystagmus

Early onset and progressive
Posterior polar subcapsular cataract

Metabolic
Diabetes mellitus*
Hypocalcaemia (primary hypoparathyroidism)
Nutritional secondary hyperparathyroidism

Nutritional
Hand rearing on milk substitutes

*Traumatic**
Blunt
Penetrating

Luxation/subluxation

Primary

Secondary
Chronic uveitis *q.v.*
Glaucoma *q.v.*
Lens shape/size abnormalities
Trauma

2.6.5   Retinal lesions

Retinal detachment

Congenital, e.g.
Collie eye anomaly
Persistent hyperplastic primary vitreous and retinal dysplasia

Iatrogenic
Complication of lens surgery

Space-occupying lesions
Extraocular
Intraocular

Systemic disease
Hypertension* *q.v.*
Severe systemic inflammatory disease
Uveodermatological syndrome
*Trauma**

Swollen optic disc

Disc oedema
    Glaucoma *q.v.*
    Post-operative hypotony
    Uveitis *q.v.*

Neoplasia
    Metastatic
    Primary

Optic neuritis
    Inflammatory
        • Granulomatous
            meningoencephalomyelitis
    Infectious
        • Blastomycosis
        • Canine distemper virus* (D)
        • Cryptococcosis
        • Histoplasmosis
        • Toxoplasmosis
    Idiopathic
    Local disease
        • Orbital abscess*
        • Orbital cellulitis*
        • Neoplasia
    Trauma*
    Toxins

Papilloedema, e.g.
    Acute glaucoma
    Hypertension *q.v.*
    Neoplasia of optic nerve
    Orbital space-occupying lesion
    Raised intracranial pressure
        • Brain tumours
        • Intracranial haemorrhage

Pseudopapilloedema
    Congenital defects

Retinal haemorrhage*, e.g.
Coagulopathy
Hypertensive retinopathy
Hyperviscosity
Inflammatory/infectious chorioretinitis
Neoplastic chorioretinitis

2.6.6 Intraocular haemorrhage/hyphaema

Chronic glaucoma

Coagulopathy

Congenital disease
Collie eye anomaly
Persistent hyaloid artery
Persistent hyperplastic primary vitreous
Vitreoretinal dysplasia

Hyperviscosity syndrome
Hyperglobulinaemia
Polycythaemia *q.v.*

Iatrogenic
Post-surgery

Inflammation, e.g.
Uveitis

Neoplasia

Neovascularisation
Retinal
Uveal

Retinal detachment q.v.

Systemic hypertension* q.v.

Trauma*

2.6.7   Abnormal appearance of anterior chamber

Anterior synechia
Anterior uveitis q.v.
Congenital lesions
Coloboma
Iris cysts
Persistent pupillary membranes

Hyphaema q.v.
Hypopyon
Deep corneal ulceration
Uveitis *q.v.*

Infiltration by neoplastic cells
Lipaemic aqueous
Masses
Foreign body*
Iris cysts
Luxated lens
Organised fibrin post inflammation*
Uveal tumours
• Adenocarcinoma
• Adenoma
• Medulloepithelioma
• Melanoma
• Metastatic

2.7   Musculoskeletal signs

2.7.1   Muscular atrophy or hypertrophy

ATROPHY

Disuse atrophy*
Orthopaedic disease* *q.v.*
Restricted exercise*

Metabolic/endocrine/systemic disease

Cachexia*
- Cardiac disease*
- Neoplasia*

Glycogen storage diseases
Hyperadrenocorticism
Hyperthyroidism* (C)
Hypothyroid myopathy (D)
Lipid storage myopathy
Mitochondrial myopathy
Poor nutritional states
- Gastrointestinal disease *q.v.*
- Inadequate protein-calorie intake

Myopathies

Degenerative/inherited

Distal myopathy of Rottweilers (D)
Fibrotic myopathy
Labrador Retriever myopathy (D)
Merosin-deficient myopathy
Muscular dystrophy
Nemaline myopathy

Inflammatory/infectious

Bacterial
Dermatomyositis
Extra-ocular myositis
Leptospirosis
Masticatory myositis
Polymyositis
Protozoal
- Neosporosis (D)
- Toxoplasmosis

Tetanus

Neurogenic

Neoplasia, e.g.
- Malignant nerve sheath tumour

Peripheral neuropathies *q.v.*
Spinal cord disease *q.v.*

HYPERTROPHY/MUSCULAR SWELLING

Athletic training*
Breed related*
Myositis ossificans
Myotonia (D)
Muscular dystrophy
Traumatic ischaemic neuromyopathy associated with bottom-hung pivot windows and garage doors (C)

2.7.2 Trismus ('lockjaw')

Drugs/toxins, e.g.

Cocaine

Inflammatory

Dermatomyositis
Granulomatous meningoencephalomyelitis
Infectious
 • Neosporosis
 • Tetanus
 • Toxoplasmosis
Masticatory myositis
Trigeminal neuritis

Mechanical

Foreign body
Malicious, e.g. placement of rubber band
Neoplasia
 • Mandibular
 • Maxillary
 • Oral
 • Orbital
 • Retrobulbar

Pain on opening jaw

Foreign body*
Myositis
Retrobulbar cellulitis or abscess*
Temporomandibular joint arthritis*

Tooth root abscess*
Trauma to buccal cavity or temporomandibular joint*

Temporomandibular joint ankylosis
Infection
Systemic arthropathies
Trauma*
Tumours

2.7.3   Weakness (see Section 1.1.8 for full listings)

Cardiovascular disease*
Endocrine disease*
Haematological disease*
Immune-mediated disease
Infectious disease*
Metabolic disease
Neuromuscular disease
Nutritional disorders
Physiological
Respiratory disease
Systemic disorders*
Drugs/toxins

2.8   Urogenital physical signs

2.8.1   Kidneys abnormal on palpation

Enlarged kidneys

Irregular surface
Feline infectious peritonitis (C)
Infarcts
Neoplasia*
Pericapsular abscess
Pericapsular haematoma
Polycystic kidney disease
Renal cyst

Smooth surface
  Acute kidney injury *q.v.*
  Amyloidosis
  Compensatory hypertrophy
  Hydronephrosis
  Neoplasia*
  Perinephric pseudocyst
  Polycystic kidney disease
  Pyelonephritis
  Pyogranulomatous nephritis
  Renal cyst

Normal-sized kidneys – irregular surface
  Infarcts
  Neoplasia*
  Pericapsular haematoma
  Polycystic kidney disease
  Renal cyst
  Subcapsular haematoma

Small kidneys

Irregular surface
  Chronic generalised glomerulo- or tubulo-interstitial disease* *q.v.*
  Hypoplastic kidneys
  Multiple infarcts

Smooth surface
  Hypoplasia

Absent kidneys
  Aplasia
  Nephrectomy

2.8.2   Bladder abnormalities

Palpable mass
  Neoplasia*
  Urolith*

Large bladder, difficult to express

Functional obstruction

Drugs/toxins, e.g.
- Atropine
- Glycopyrronium bromide
- Propantheline bromide
- Tricyclic antidepressants

Neurological disease
- Upper motor neurone bladder*
    - Spinal disorders cranial to L7 *q.v.*

Psychogenic*
- Pain
- Stress

Reflex dyssynergia

Mechanical obstruction

Matrix-crystalline plugs*
Neoplasia*
- Bladder
- Urethra

Prostatomegaly*
Urethral stricture
Uroliths*
- Bladder neck
- Urethra

Large bladder, easy to express

Normal

Neurological disease, e.g.

Dysautonomia
Lower motor neurone bladder*
- Cauda equina syndrome
- Lesion of sacral spinal cord
- Lesions of pelvic/lumbosacral plexus

Small/difficult to palpate bladder

Congenital hypoplasia
Ectopic ureters
Non-distensible bladder

- Diffuse bladder-wall neoplasia
- Severe cystitis, e.g.
  - Calculi
  - Infection
  - Trauma

Oliguric/anuric kidney injury *q.v.*
Recent voiding*
Ruptured bladder
Ruptured ureters

2.8.3   Prostate abnormal on palpation

Enlargement

Diffuse

   Bacterial prostatitis
   Benign prostatic hyperplasia*
   Neoplasia

Focal lesions

   Abscess
   Cysts
- Paraprostatic
- Prostatic

   Neoplasia

2.8.4   Uterus abnormal on palpation

Enlargement on palpation

   Haemometra
   Hydrometra
   Mucometra
   Neoplasia*
- Adenocarcinoma
- Adenoma
- Leiomyoma
- Leiomyosarcoma

   Post partum*
   Pregnancy*
   Pyometra*

2.8.5 Testicular abnormalities

Single palpable testis

Castration of single descended testis with subsequent descent
of unilateral cryptorchid testis
Unilateral cryptorchid*
Unilateral testicular agenesis

No palpable testis

Bilateral cryptorchid*
Bilateral testicular agenesis
Intersex abnormalities
Previous castration*

Large testis

Acute infection
Inguinoscrotal hernia
Neoplasia
Sperm granuloma
Testicular torsion

Small testis

Chronic inflammation
Cryptorchidism
Degeneration
Hypoplasia
Intersex
Sertoli cell tumour in contralateral testis

2.8.6 Penis abnormalities

Paraphimosis

Chronic balanoposthitis
Foreign bodies in prepuce
Fracture of the os penis
Idiopathic
Obstruction of the preputial opening by long hair*

Small preputial opening
- Congenital
- Post-surgical
- Traumatic

Soft tissue trauma*
Spinal lesions

Penile bleeding

Haematuria* *q.v.*
Herpes virus
Transmissible venereal tumour
Other tumours (benign polypoid to variety malignant)
Trauma

Prostatic disease, e.g.
Benign hyperplasia

Urethral disease, e.g.
Urethral prolapse

PART 3
RADIOGRAPHIC AND ULTRASONOGRAPHIC SIGNS

3.1 Thoracic radiography

3.1.1 Artefactual causes of increased lung opacity

Chemical stains/dirty cassettes
Dirty or wet fur
Forelimbs not pulled sufficiently forwards
Movement blur
Obesity
Poorly inflated lungs
- Abdominal distension
- Expiratory film
- Upper airway obstruction
Underdevelopment
Underexposure

3.1.2 Increased bronchial pattern

Normal variation*
Chondrodystrophic breeds
Older dogs

Differential Diagnosis in Small Animal Medicine, Second Edition.
Alex Gough and Kate Murphy.
© 2015 John Wiley & Sons, Ltd. Published 2015 by John Wiley & Sons, Ltd.

Bronchial wall oedema, e.g.
Congestive heart failure*

Bronchiectasis
Chronic bronchitis*
Primary ciliary dyskinesia (D)

Endocrine
Hyperadrenocorticism

Infection
Bacterial*
Fungal, e.g.
- *Pneumocystis carinii*
Parasitic, e.g.
- *Crenosoma vulpis* (D)
Protozoal, e.g.
- Toxoplasmosis
Viral

Inflammation, e.g.
Eosinophilic bronchopneumopathy (pulmonary infiltrate with eosinophilia) (D)
Feline asthma (C)
Idiopathic

Neoplasia
Bronchogenic carcinoma
Lymphoma

3.1.3   Increased alveolar pattern

Atelectasis
Airway obstruction
Chronic pleural or pulmonary disease*
Collapse of the lung lobes under general anaesthesia*
Extra-pulmonary thoracic mass
Feline asthma* (C)
Lack of surfactant (newborn, acute respiratory distress syndrome)

Lung lobe torsion
Pleural effusion* *q.v.*
Pneumothorax* *q.v.*
Recumbency

Inflammation/immune mediated
Eosinophilic bronchopneumopathy (pulmonary infiltrate with eosinophilia)

Neoplasia
Malignant histiocytosis
Primary lung tumour, e.g.
• Bronchoalveolar carcinoma
Pulmonary lymphomatoid granulomatosis

Pneumonia
Aspiration pneumonia
Aspirated foreign body*
Aspirated secretions
Cleft palate
Gastrobronchial fistula
Generalised weakness
Iatrogenic, e.g.
• Anaesthetic complication
• Force feeding
• Incorrectly placed stomach tube
Oesophagotracheal/bronchial fistula
Regurgitation, e.g.
• Megaoesophagus
Swallowing disorders
Vomiting

Bronchopneumonia, e.g.
Canine distemper virus with secondary bacterial infection* (D)
Tracheobronchitis*

Bacterial, e.g.
Tuberculosis
Tularaemia

Fungal, e.g.
Pneumocystis carinii

Parasitic, e.g.
Aelurostrongylus abstrusus (C)
Angiostrongylus vasorum (D)
Dirofilaria immitis
Oslerus osleri (D)

Miscellaneous
Kartagener's syndrome
Primary ciliary dyskinesia
Radiation therapy

Pulmonary haemorrhage
Coagulopathy *q.v.*
Exercise induced
Idiopathic
Neoplasia*
Trauma*

Pulmonary oedema
Acute dyspnoea in Swedish hunting dogs
Acute pancreatitis*
Airway obstruction
Brain trauma
Congestive heart failure*
Electrocution
Hypoalbuminaemia
Hypostatic congestion*
Iatrogenic
 • Aspirated hypertonic contrast media
 • IV contrast media
 • Over-hydration
Inhalation of irritant gases/smoke
Lung lobe torsion
Near drowning
Obstruction of pulmonary drainage
mechanisms, e.g.
 • Hilar mass
Post-ictal

Re-expansion, e.g.
- Post pneumothorax

Seizures

Other CNS disease

Uraemia *q.v.*

Acute respiratory distress syndrome

Iatrogenic, e.g.
- Over-hydration
- Oxygen therapy

Infection

Inhalation pneumonia

Pancreatitis

Trauma

Toxins

Alpha-napthylthiourea

Endotoxin

Ethylene glycol

Paracetamol

Snake venom

Pulmonary thromboembolism

3.1.4 Increased interstitial pattern

Nodular

Artefact

End-on view of blood vessels

Nipples

Objects adhering to coat

Ossification of costochondral junctions

Thoracic wall nodules

Infection

Abscesses

Feline infectious peritonitis* (C)

Granulomata
- Bacterial
- Foreign body*
- Fungal

Hydatid cysts

Parasitic
- *Aelurostrongylus abstrusus* (C)
- *Crenosoma vulpis* (D)
- *Oslerus osleri* (D)
- *Paragonimus kellicotti* (D)
- Tularaemia
- Visceral larva migrans

Pneumonia
- Fungal pneumonia
- Haematogenous bacterial pneumonia
- Mycobacterial pneumonia

Protozoal, e.g.
- Toxoplasmosis

Neoplasia

Lymphoma*

Metastatic tumours*

Primary lung tumours

Miscellaneous

Calcified pleural plaques*

Disseminated intravascular coagulation

Haematomata

Idiopathic mineralisation

Pulmonary osteomata
(heterotopic bone)*

Diffuse/unstructured

Artefact, e.g.

Expiratory film

Neoplasia

Oedema (early) *q.v.*

Drugs/toxins

Chronic glucocorticoid administration

Paraquat

Endocrine
  Hyperadrenocorticism

Infection
  Bacterial
  Fungal, e.g.
  - Blastomycosis
  - Coccidioidomycosis
  - Cryptococcosis
  - Histoplasmosis
  - *Pneumocystis carinii* (D)

  Mycoplasmosis
  Parasitic
  - *Aelurostrongylus abstrusus* (C)
  - *Angiostrongylus vasorum* (D)
  - Babesiosis
  - Dirofilariasis

  Protozoal, e.g.
  Rickettsial, e.g.
  - Rocky Mountain spotted fever (D)

  Toxoplasmosis
  Viral, e.g.
  - Canine distemper virus* (D)
  - Feline infectious peritonitis* (C)

Inhalation
  Dust
  Irritant gases

Miscellaneous

  Acute respiratory distress syndrome
  Pancreatitis
  Pulmonary thromboembolism
  Radiation therapy
  Uraemia* *q.v.*
  Very old animals
  Very young animals

Pulmonary fibrosis
  Idiopathic
  Secondary to chronic respiratory disease

Pulmonary haemorrhage
    Coagulopathy *q.v.*
    Exercise induced
    Idiopathic
    Neoplasia
    Trauma

Reticular pattern
    Normal ageing*
    Chronic fibrosis
    Fungal pneumonia
    Lymphoma*
    Metastatic neoplasia*

3.1.5   Increased vascular pattern

Increased size of pulmonary arteries
    Aelurostrongylus abstrusus (C)
    Angiostrongylus vasorum (D)
    Dirofilariasis
    Large left-to-right shunts, e.g.
      • Atrial septal defect
      • Endocardial cushion defects
      • Patent ductus arteriosus
      • Ventricular septal defect
    Pulmonary hypertension
    Pulmonary thromboembolism

Increased size of pulmonary veins
    Left-sided heart failure*
    Left-to-right shunts, in some cases

Increased size of pulmonary arteries and veins
    Left-to-right shunts, e.g.
      • Atrial septal defect
      • Endocardial cushion defects
      • Patent ductus arteriosus
      • Ventricular septal defect

3.1.6 Decreased vascular pattern

Generalised

Pericardial disease, e.g.
Pericardial effusion* *q.v.*
Restrictive pericarditis

Pulmonary hypoperfusion
Hypoadrenocorticism (D)
Localised hypoperfusion due to pulmonary thromboembolism
Pulmonic stenosis
Severe dehydration*
Shock*
Tetralogy of Fallot

Pulmonary overinflation
Air trapping
- Chronic bronchitis* (D)
- Feline asthma* (C)
- Upper respiratory tract obstruction, e.g.
  - Foreign body*
  - Nasopharyngeal polyp* (C)
Compensatory
- Following lobectomy
- Secondary to atelectasis of another lobe
- Secondary to congenital lobar atresia/agenesis
Emphysema
Iatrogenic
- Anaesthesia

Right-to-left cardiac shunts, e.g.
Atrial septal defect
Reverse-shunting patent ductus arteriosus
Tetralogy of Fallot
Ventricular septal defect

Localised
Emphysema
Pulmonary thromboembolism

3.1.7　Cardiac diseases that may be associated with a normal cardiac silhouette

Bacterial endocarditis
Congestive heart failure overzealously treated with diuretics
Constrictive pericarditis
Functional murmurs*
Hypertrophic cardiomyopathy* (C)
Neoplasia
Small atrial septal defect
Small ventricular septal defect

3.1.8　Increased size of cardiac silhouette

Generalised cardiomegaly

Normal variation, e.g.
Greyhound*
Artefact
Bacterial endocarditis
Bradycardia* *q.v.*
Chronic anaemia* *q.v.*
Concurrent mitral and tricuspid valve deficiency
Dysplasia
Intrapericardial fat
Mediastinal fat
Myxomatous degeneration* (D)
Congenital cardiac disease, e.g.
　• Peritoneopericardial diaphragmatic hernia
Enlargement of specific chamber sizes *q.v.*
Pericardial effusion* *q.v.*

Myocardial disease

Inflammatory
　• Immune mediated, e.g. rheumatoid arthritis
　• Infectious, e.g.
　　◦ Bacterial
　　◦ Fungal
　　◦ Parvovirus
　　◦ Protozoal

Ischaemic
- Arteriosclerosis

Noninflammatory
- Dilated cardiomyopathy*
- Hypertrophic cardiomyopathy (C)*
- Restrictive cardiomyopathy (C)

Secondary
- Acromegaly
- Amyloidosis
- End-stage mitral valve insufficiency* (D)
- Glycogen storage disease
- Hypertension* *q.v.*
- Hyperthyroidism* (C)
- Mucopolysaccharidosis
- Neoplasia
- Neuromuscular disease
- Nutrition
  - l-Carnitine deficiency
  - Taurine deficiency
- Trauma
- Drugs/toxins
  - Doxorubicin
  - Heavy metals

Volume overload

Iatrogenic
Left-sided heart failure
- Bacterial endocarditis
- Dilated cardiomyopathy*
- Mitral valve dysplasia
- Myxomatous degeneration
  of the mitral valve* (D)

3.1.9 Decreased size of cardiac silhouette

Atrophic myopathies
Constrictive pericarditis
Hypoadrenocorticism (D)
Post thoracotomy

Artefact
> Deep-chested dogs
> Deep inspiration
> Heart displaced from sternum, e.g.
> - Mediastinal shift
> - Pneumothorax
> Pulmonary overinflation, e.g.
> - Emphysema
> - Hyperventilation

Decrease in muscle mass
> Chronic systemic disease
> Malnutrition
> Myopathies

Shock* q.v., e.g.
> Hypovolaemia, e.g.
> - Blood loss
> - Severe dehydration

3.1.10 Abnormalities of the ribs

Congenital disorders
> Absence of the xiphisternum
> Agenesis/hypoplasia of the 13th rib*
> Pectus excavatum
> Supernumerary ribs

New bone
> Cartilaginous exostoses
> Healed fractures
> Mineralisation of the costal cartilages*
> Neoplasia
> Non-union fractures
> Periosteal reaction to soft tissue mass

Osteolysis
> Metastatic tumours
> Osteomyelitis
> Primary tumours

- Chondrosarcoma
- Fibrosarcoma
- Haemangiosarcoma
- Multiple myeloma
- Osteoma
- Osteosarcoma

Thoracic wall trauma*

3.1.11 Abnormalities of the oesophagus

OESOPHAGEAL DILATATION
Generalised

Acquired megaoesophagus
Idiopathic
Immune-mediated neuromuscular disease
- Myasthenia gravis
- Polymyositis
- Polyradiculoneuritis
- Systemic lupus erythematosus
Metabolic/endocrine
- Hypoadrenocorticism (D)
- Hypothyroidism* (D)
Miscellaneous
- Dysautonomia
- Gastric dilatation/volvulus*
- Hypertrophic muscular dystrophy
- Oesophageal foreign body
- Reflux oesophagitis
- Thiamine deficiency
Toxic
- Botulinum toxin
- Chlorinated hydrocarbons
- Heavy metals
- Herbicides
- Organophosphates
- Snake venom
- Tetanus

Congenital megaoesophagus
    Canine giant axonal neuropathy (D)
    Glycogen storage disease
    Hereditary megaoesophagus
    Hereditary myopathy
    Vascular ring anomaly, e.g.
- Double aortic arch
- Normal aorta with aberrant right subclavian artery
- Persistent right aortic arch
- Persistent right ductus arteriosus
- Right aortic arch with aberrant right subclavian artery

Transient megaoesophagus
    Hiatal hernia
    Respiratory infection
    Sedation/anaesthesia*

Localised
    Redundant oesophagus

Acquired
    Dilatation cranial to a gastro-oesophageal intussusception
    Dilatation cranial to acquired stricture, e.g.
- Extraluminal compression
- Granuloma
- Mucosal adhesion
- Neoplasia
- Post general anaesthesia

    Dilatation cranial to an oesophageal foreign body*
    Oesophagitis
    Scar tissue post trauma

Congenital
    Dilatation cranial to a congenital stenosis
    Dilatation cranial to oesophageal hiatal hernia
    Segmental oesophageal hypomotility
    Vascular ring anomaly, e.g.
- Double aortic arch
- Normal aorta with aberrant right subclavian artery

- Persistent right aortic arch
- Persistent right ductus arteriosus
- Right aortic arch with aberrant right subclavian artery
- Oesophageal diverticulum

Transient
   Aerophagia*
   Dyspnoea*
   Swallowing*

INCREASED OESOPHAGEAL OPACITY

Bony density
   Foreign body*
   Megaoesophagus with collection of food
   Osteosarcoma, e.g.
- Secondary to *Spirocerca lupi* (D)

Soft tissue density
   Megaoesophagus with collection of food/water
   Normal variation, e.g.
- Fluid in the oesophagus*
- Superimposition of the trachea*

Soft tissue mass
   Intraluminal
- Food-containing oesophageal diverticulum
- Foreign body*
- Gastro-oesophageal intussusception
- Oesophageal hiatal hernia

   Intramural
- Abscess
- Foreign body
- Granuloma, e.g.
  - *Spirocerca lupi* (D)
- Neoplasia
  - *Metastatic*
  - *Primary oesophageal, e.g.*
    Leiomyoma/sarcoma

Squamous cell carcinoma
- Secondary to *Spirocerca lupi* (D)

Extraluminal
- Abscess
- Neoplasia
- Paraoesophageal hiatal hernia

3.1.12 Abnormalities of the trachea

Dorsal displacement
Artefact
- Expiration
- Rotation
- Ventroflexion

Breed variation*
Cardiomegaly*
Cranioventral mediastinal mass
Heart base tumour
Tracheobronchial lymphadenopathy*

Ventral displacement
Craniodorsal mediastinal mass
Megaoesophagus
Oesophageal foreign body*
Post-stenotic aortic dilatation
Vertebral spondylosis

Lateral displacement
Artefact
- Expiration
- Rotation
- Ventroflexion

Breed variation*
Cranial mediastinal mass
Heart base tumour
Mediastinal shift *q.v.*
Megaoesophagus
Vascular ring anomaly

Narrowing
Congenital hypoplasia

Artefact
Hyperextension of the neck
Superimposition of the
muscle/oesophagus

External compression
Cranial mediastinal mass
Megaoesophagus
Oesophageal foreign body*
Vascular ring anomaly

Mucosal thickening
Feline infectious peritonitis* (C)
Inflammation, e.g.
  • Allergy*
  • Infection*
  • Irritant gases
Submucosal haemorrhage, e.g.
  • Coagulopathy

Stricture/stenosis
Congenital
Excessive pressure from the cuff
of endotracheal tube
Focal intramural mass
Post-traumatic injury

Tracheal collapse *
Acquired, e.g.
  • Secondary to chronic bronchitis
Congenital

Opacification of the lumen
Abscess
Aspiration of positive contrast agents
Foreign body*
Granuloma
Oslerus osleri
Polyp

Neoplasia
　Adenocarcinoma
　Chondrosarcoma
　Leiomyoma
　Lymphoma
　Mast cell tumour
　Osteochondroma
　Osteosarcoma

3.1.13　Pleural effusion

Bile pleuritis
Ruptured biliary tree with diaphragmatic hernia

Blood
Autoimmune disorders, e.g.
* Immune-mediated thrombocytopenia
Angiostrongylus vasorum infection
Coagulopathy
Neoplasia, e.g.
* Haemangiosarcoma
Trauma

Chyle
Congenital duct malformation (D)
Constrictive pleuritis
Cranial mediastinal mass
Diaphragmatic rupture*
Feline dirofilariasis (C)
Idiopathic*
Lung lobe torsion
Neoplasia
Peritoneopericardial diaphragmatic hernia
Post pacemaker implantation (C)
Rupture of the thoracic duct

Heart disease
Dilated cardiomyopathy (C)
Hypertrophic cardiomyopathy (C)*

Pericardial disease
Right-sided heart failure (C)

Obstruction of the thoracic duct
Intraluminal
- Granuloma
- Neoplasia
Extraluminal
- Increased intrathoracic pressure

Exudate

Actinomycosis
Autoimmune disorders, e.g.
- Rheumatoid arthritis
- Systemic lupus erythematosus
Feline infectious peritonitis* (C)
Fungal infection
Neoplasia*
Nocardiosis
Pneumonia*
Pyothorax*
- Extension from pulmonary parenchymal lesion
Foreign body
- Haematogenous spread
- Penetrating thoracic wound
- Penetration of the trachea/oesophagus
Tuberculosis

Transudate/modified transudate

Congestive heart failure*
Diaphragmatic rupture*
Foreign body
Hyperthyroidism* (C)
Hypoproteinaemia *q.v.**
- Liver disease*
- Protein-losing enteropathy*
- Protein-losing nephropathy*
Idiopathic
Lung lobe torsion

Neoplasia, e.g.
- Lymphoma*
Pancreatitis
Pneumonia*
Thromboembolism

3.1.14 Pneumothorax

Artefact
Overdevelopment
Overexposure*
Overinflation of the lungs
Skin folds*
Undercirculation

Iatrogenic
Cardiopulmonary resuscitation
Leaking chest drain
Lung aspiration/biopsy
Thoracocentesis
Thoracotomy

Spontaneous
Bacterial pneumonia
Parasites
- Dirofilariasis
- *Oslerus osleri*
- *Paragonimus*
Pleural adhesions
Rupture of congenital or acquired bullae,
cysts or blebs
Tumours*

Trauma
Perforation of the lung*
Perforation of the oesophagus
Perforation of the thoracic wall*
Perforation of the trachea/bronchi*

3.1.15 Abnormalities of the diaphragm

Cranial displacement
Diaphragmatic rupture/hernia*

Abdominal causes
Abdominal neoplasia*
Ascites*
Gastric dilatation*
Obesity*
Organomegaly*, e.g.
- Liver
- Spleen
Pneumoperitoneum
Pregnancy*
Pyometra*

Thoracic causes
Atelectasis
Diaphragmatic paralysis
Diaphragmatic tumour
Expiratory film*
Lung lobectomy
Pleural adhesions
Pulmonary fibrosis

Caudal displacement

Abdominal causes
Abdominal body wall rupture/hernia leading to abdominal organ displacement
Poor body condition

Thoracic causes
Chronic dyspnoea*
Deep inspiration*
Intrathoracic mass*
Pleural effusion*
Pneumothorax*

Irregular diaphragmatic contour

Diaphragmatic rupture/hernia*
Hypertrophic muscular dystrophy
Pleural masses, e.g.
- Granuloma
- Neoplasia

Severe lung hyperinflation

Lack of visualisation of diaphragmatic border

Artefact, e.g.
- Expiratory film

Diaphragmatic hernia*
Increased lung density, e.g.
- Alveolar pattern*

Neoplasia adjacent to diaphragm*
Peritoneopericardial diaphragmatic hernia
Pleural effusion*

3.1.16   Mediastinal abnormalities

Mediastinal masses

Aortic aneurysm
Cyst
Granuloma
- Actinomycosis
- Nocardiosis

Haematoma
Hiatal hernia
Oesophageal dilatation
Oesophageal foreign body*
Oesophageal granuloma
- *Spirocerca lupi (D)*

Thymus

Artefact

Left or right atrial enlargement
Lung lobe tip

Pleural fluid
Post-stenotic dilatation of the aorta or pulmonary artery

Lymphadenopathy
  Bacterial
  - Actinomycosis
  - Nocardiosis
  - Tuberculosis
  Eosinophilic pulmonary granulomatosis
  Fungal
  - Blastomycosis
  - Coccidioidomycosis
  - Cryptococcosis
  - Histoplasmosis
  Neoplasia
  - Lymphoma*
  - Malignant histiocytosis
  - Metastatic neoplasia*

Neoplasia
  Ectopic parathyroid tumour
  Ectopic thyroid tumour
  Fibrosarcoma
  Heart base tumours
  Lipoma*
  Lymphoma*
  Malignant histiocytosis
  Rib tumour
  Thymoma

Mediastinal shift

Away from affected hemithorax
  Diaphragmatic rupture/hernia*
  Lobar emphysema
  Lung mass*
  Oblique view
  Pleural mass*
  Unilateral pleural effusion*
  Unilateral pneumothorax*

Towards affected hemithorax
  Atelectasis
  - Feline asthma* (C)
  - Foreign body*
  - Mass*
  - Radiation
  Hypostatic congestion*, e.g.
  - General anaesthesia
  - Illness resulting in prolonged lateral recumbency
  Lobar agenesis/hypoplasia
  Lobectomy
  Lung lobe torsion
  Oblique view
  Radiation-induced fibrosis
  Unilateral phrenic nerve paralysis

Pneumomediastinum
  Emphysematous mediastinitis
  Iatrogenic
  Secondary to severe dyspnoea*

Air from neck
  Gas-forming bacteria
  Trauma*, e.g.
  - Jugular venepuncture
  - Oesophagus
  - Pharynx
  - Soft tissue
  - Trachea

Air from bronchi/lungs, e.g.
  Lung lobe torsion
  Spontaneous
  Trauma*

Widened mediastinum
  Normal variation*
  - Bulldogs
  Abscess
  - Foreign body

Masses (see succeeding text)
Megaoesophagus *q.v.*
Obesity*

Mediastinal effusions, e.g.
Chylomediastinum
Haemorrhage
- Coagulopathy
- Neoplasia
- Trauma*

Mediastinitis/mediastinal abscess
Feline infectious peritonitis (C)
Lymphadenitis
Oesophageal/tracheal perforation
Penetrating neck wound*
Pleuritis*
Pneumonia*

Oedema*
Congestive heart failure*
Hypoproteinaemia* *q.v.*
Neoplasia*
Trauma*

3.2 Abdominal radiography

3.2.1 Liver

Focal enlargement

Infection/inflammation
Abscess
Granuloma

Miscellaneous
Biliary pseudocyst
Cyst

Haematoma
Hepatic arteriovenous fistula
Hyperplastic/regenerative nodule*
Liver lobe torsion

*Neoplasia**
Biliary cystadenoma
Haemangiosarcoma
Hepatocellular carcinoma*
Hepatoma
Lymphoma*
Malignant histiocytosis
Metastatic*

Generalised enlargement

Endocrine disease
Acromegaly
Diabetes mellitus*
Hyperadrenocorticism

Infection/inflammation
Abscess
Feline infectious peritonitis* (C)
Fungal infection
Granuloma
Hepatitis*
Lymphocytic cholangitis*

Neoplasia, e.g.

Haemangiosarcoma
Lymphoma*
Malignant histiocytosis
Mast cell infiltration (mastocytosis/mast cell tumour)
Metastatic tumours*

Venous congestion
Caudal vena cava occlusion (post caval syndrome)
- Adhesions
- Cardiac neoplasia
- Congenital cardiac disease

- Diaphragmatic rupture/hernia*
- Dirofilariasis
- Pericardial disease
- Thoracic mass
- Thrombosis
- Trauma*

Right-sided congestive heart failure, e.g.
- Dilated cardiomyopathy*
- Pericardial disease, e.g. pericardial effusion *q.v.*
- Tricuspid regurgitation

Miscellaneous
Amyloidosis
Cholestasis *q.v.**
Cirrhosis (early)*
Hepatic lipidosis (C)
Nodular hyperplasia*
Storage diseases

Drugs
Glucocorticoids

Reduced liver size

Breed variation (e.g. apparent microhepatica in deep-chested dogs)
Cirrhosis
Diaphragmatic rupture/hernia*
Hypoadrenocorticism (D)
Idiopathic hepatic fibrosis
Portosystemic shunt
- Acquired
- Congenital

3.2.2 Spleen

Enlargement

Normal, e.g.
Breed related*

Congestion
  Gastric dilatation/volvulus*
  Portal hypertension
  Right-sided congestive heart failure
  Sedation and general anaesthesia*
  Splenic thrombosis
  Splenic torsion

Haematoma*
  Idiopathic
  Secondary to neoplasia
  Trauma

Hyperplasia*
  Chronic anaemia *q.v.*
  Chronic infection
  Lymphoid

Inflammation/immune mediated
  Hypereosinophilic syndrome
  Immune-mediated haemolytic anaemia
  Systemic lupus erythematosus

Infection
  Abscess
  Babesiosis
  Bacteraemia
  Ehrlichiosis
  Feline infectious peritonitis* (C)
  Fungal infections
  Infectious canine hepatitis (D)
  Leishmaniasis
  Mycobacteria
  Mycoplasma
  Toxoplasmosis
  Salmonellosis
  Septicaemia*

Neoplasia
  Fibrosarcoma
  Haemangioma

Haemangiosarcoma*
Leiomyosarcoma
Leukaemia
Lymphoma*
Malignant histiocytosis
Multiple myeloma
Systemic mastocytosis

Miscellaneous

Amyloidosis
Extramedullary haematopoiesis*
Infarction
Splenic myeloid metaplasia

Trauma
Foreign body
Penetrating wound

Reduction in size

Dehydration*
Shock* *q.v.*

Absence

Artefact
Displacement through hernia/rupture
Splenectomy

3.2.3 Stomach

Abnormal contents

Gas
Aerophagia*
Gastric dilatation/volvulus*

Mineral opacity
Foreign body*
Gravel sign (outflow obstruction)*

Iatrogenic
- Barium
- Bismuth
- Kaolin

Soft tissue opacity
Blood clot
Food/ingested liquid*
Foreign body*
Intussusception
Neoplasia
Polyp

Caudal displacement
Enlargement of the thoracic cavity, e.g.
- Overinflation of the lungs
- Pleural effusion* *q.v.*
Hepatomegaly* *q.v.*

Cranial displacement
Diaphragmatic hernia/rupture*
Hiatal hernia
Late pregnancy*
Microhepatica
Neoplasia/mass, e.g.
- Colonic
- Mesenteric
- Pancreatic
Peritoneopericardial
diaphragmatic hernia

Delayed gastric emptying
Gastritis*
General anaesthesia/sedation*

Functional disorders
Adynamic ileus*
Dysautonomia
Pancreatitis*
Primary dysmotilities
Uraemia* *q.v.*

Pyloric outflow obstruction
    Chronic hyperplastic gastropathy
    Fibrosis/scar tissue
    Foreign body*
    Granuloma
    Neoplasia
        • Biliary
        • Duodenal
        • Gastric
        • Pancreatic
    Pyloric hypertrophy
        • Mucosal
        • Muscular
    Ulceration

Pylorospasm
    Anxiety
    Stress

Ulceration
    Duodenal
    Gastric

Distended
    Acute gastritis*
    Gastric dilatation volvulus*
    Pancreatitis*

Aerophagia*
    Bolting food
    Dyspnoea
    Pain

Iatrogenic
    Anticholinergic drugs
    Endoscopic inflation
    Misplaced endotracheal tube
    Stomach tube

Outflow obstruction
    Fibrosis/scarring
    Foreign body*

Granuloma
Muscular or mucosal hypertrophy
Neoplasia
Pylorospasm
Ulceration

Increased wall thickness (contrast radiography)

Diffuse
Inflammation
- Chronic gastritis*
- Eosinophilic gastritis*

Neoplasia
- Lymphoma
- Pancreatic tumour

Chronic hyperplastic gastropathy

Focal
Artefact
- Empty stomach

Hypertrophy
- Mucosal
- Muscular

Inflammation
- Eosinophilic
- Fungal infection
- Granulomatous

Neoplasia
- Adenocarcinoma
- Leiomyoma
- Leiomyosarcoma
- Lymphoma

3.2.4   Intestines

SMALL INTESTINE

Bunching

Adhesions*
Linear foreign body*
Obesity*

Displacement

Caudal displacement
Distended stomach*
Empty urinary bladder*
Hepatomegaly* *q.v.*
Hernias*
- Inguinal*
- Perineal*

Cranial displacement
Empty stomach*
Enlarged urinary bladder* *q.v.*
Enlarged uterus*
- Pregnancy*
- Pyometra*
Microhepatica

Diaphragmatic disorders
Peritoneopericardial diaphragmatic hernia
Rupture/hernia*

Lateral displacement
Hepatomegaly* *q.v.*
Prolonged lateral recumbency*
Renomegaly* *q.v.*
Splenomegaly* *q.v.*

Increased width of small intestinal loops

Artefact
Mistaking colon for small intestine

Functional obstruction
Dysautonomia
Electrolyte imbalances* *q.v.*
Pancreatitis*
Peritonitis*
Recent abdominal surgery*
Secondary to chronic mechanical obstruction*
Severe gastroenteritis*

Mechanical obstruction
   Abscess
   Adhesions*
   Caecal impaction
   Constipation*
   Foreign body*
   Granuloma
   Intestinal volvulus
   Intussusception
   Neoplasia, e.g.
- Adenocarcinoma
- Leiomyoma
- Leiomyosarcoma
- Lymphoma

   Polyps
   Strangulation in hernia/mesenteric tear
   Stricture

Variation in small intestinal contents

Bony/mineral density
   Food*
   Foreign body*
   Iatrogenic
- Contrast media
- Medications

Fluid/soft tissue density
   Normal*
   Diffuse infiltrative neoplasia
   Functional obstruction
- Dysautonomia
- Electrolyte imbalances* *q.v.*
- Pancreatitis*
- Peritonitis*
- Recent abdominal surgery*
- Secondary to chronic mechanical obstruction*
- Severe gastroenteritis*

   Mechanical obstruction
- Abscess
- Adhesions*

- Caecal impaction
- Constipation*
- Foreign body*
- Granuloma
- Intestinal volvulus
- Intussusception
- Neoplasia, e.g.
  - Adenocarcinoma
  - Leiomyoma
  - Leiomyosarcoma
  - Lymphoma
- Polyps
- Strangulation in hernia/mesenteric tear

Mistaking colon or enlarged uterus for small intestine

Gas density

Normal*

Adhesions*

Aerophagia*

Enteritis*

Functional obstruction

- Dysautonomia
- Electrolyte imbalances* *q.v.*
- Pancreatitis*
- Peritonitis*
- Recent abdominal surgery*
- Secondary to chronic mechanical obstruction*
- Severe gastroenteritis*

Mechanical obstruction

- Abscess
- Adhesions
- Caecal impaction
- Constipation*
- Foreign body*
- Granuloma
- Intestinal volvulus
- Intussusception
- Neoplasia, e.g.
  - Adenocarcinoma
  - Leiomyoma

- Leiomyosarcoma
- Lymphoma
- Polyps
- Strangulation in hernia/mesenteric tear

Partial obstruction*
Prolonged recumbency*

Delayed intestinal transit time

Diffuse neoplasia
Enteritis*
Inflammatory bowel disease*
Sedation/general anaesthesia*

Functional obstruction

Dysautonomia
Electrolyte imbalances* *q.v.*
Pancreatitis*
Peritonitis*
Recent abdominal surgery*
Secondary to chronic mechanical obstruction*
Severe gastroenteritis*

Mechanical obstruction (partial)

Abscess
Adhesions*
Caecal impaction
Constipation*
Foreign body*
Granuloma
Intussusception
Neoplasia, e.g.
- Adenocarcinoma
- Leiomyoma
- Leiomyosarcoma
- Lymphoma

Polyps
Strangulation in hernia/mesenteric tear

Luminal filling defects on contrast radiography

Foreign body*
Intussusception

Neoplasia
Parasitism*
Polyp
Ulcer

Increased wall thickness (contrast radiography)

Inflammatory bowel disease*
Fungal infections
Lymphangiectasia
Neoplasia, e.g.
- Adenocarcinoma
- Leiomyoma
- Leiomyosarcoma
- Lymphoma

LARGE INTESTINE

Dilatation

Constipation/obstipation* *q.v.*

Displacement

Ascending colon
Adrenal mass
Duodenal dilatation*
Hepatomegaly* *q.v.*
Lymphadenopathy* *q.v.*
Pancreatic mass
Renomegaly *q.v.*

Transverse colon
Diaphragmatic rupture/hernia*
Dilatation of the stomach*
Enlarged bladder* *q.v.*
Enlarged uterus*
Hepatomegaly* *q.v.*
Lymphadenopathy* *q.v.*
Microhepatica *q.v.*
Mid-abdominal mass*
Pancreatic mass

Descending colon
  Adrenal mass
  Enlarged bladder* *q.v.*
  Enlarged uterus* *q.v.*
  Hepatomegaly* *q.v.*
  Lymphadenopathy* *q.v.*
  Prostatomegaly*
  Renomegaly* *q.v.*
  Retroperitoneal fluid
  Splenomegaly* *q.v.*

Rectum
  Paraprostatic cyst
  Perineal hernia*
  Prostatomegaly*
  Sacral or vertebral mass
  Urethral mass
  Vaginal mass
  Other pelvic/intrapelvic mass

Variation in contents

Empty
  Normal
  Caecal inversion
  Enema
  Gastric/small intestinal obstruction* *q.v.*
  Large intestinal diarrhoea* *q.v.*
  Intussusception
  Neoplasia
  Typhlitis

Soft tissue/mineral density
  Caecal impaction
  Constipation/obstipation* *q.v.*
  Undigested dietary material*

Increased wall thickness (contrast radiography)
  Colitis*
  Fibrosis from previous trauma/surgery
  Neoplasia

Luminal filling defects on contrast radiography

Caecal inversion
Faeces*
Foreign body*
Intussusception
Masses
- Neoplasia
- Polyps

3.2.5 Ureters

Dilated

Ascending infection
Ectopic ureter
- Congenital
- Ureteral obstruction, e.g. ligation
External compression, e.g.
- Abdominal mass*
Hydroureter
- Iatrogenic
- Neoplasia
- Stricture following ureterolith or other trauma
- Ureterolith

Ureteral diverticula

Ureterocoele

3.2.6 Bladder

Abnormal bladder contents (contrast cystography)

Filling defects

Artefact
Air bubbles*
Blood clots*
Calculi*
Neoplasia
Polyps
Severe cystitis*

Increased opacity
  Blood clots*
  Neoplasia
  Polyps
  Uroliths*

Abnormal shape
  Diverticula
  Herniation
  Neoplasia
  Patent urachus
  Positioning errors
  Rupture

Displacement
  Abdominal hernia/rupture*
  Constipation/obstipation* *q.v.*
  Enlarged uterus* *q.v.*
  Lymphadenopathy* *q.v.*
  Obesity*
  Perineal hernia*
  Prepubic tendon rupture
  Prostatomegaly*
  Short urethra
  Traumatic urethral injury

Failure of the bladder to distend (contrast radiography)
  Congenital defects, e.g.
  Ectopic ureters
  Hypoplasia
  Cystitis*
  Neoplasia
  Rupture

Enlarged bladder
  Normal*

Functional obstruction
  Neurological
  • Cauda equina syndrome
  • Dysautonomia

- Upper motor neurone spinal cord lesion *q.v.*, e.g.
  - Intervertebral disc disease* (D)
  - Trauma
  - Tumour

Psychogenic*
- Lack of outside/litter access
- Pain
- Stress

Mechanical obstruction

Crystalline–matrix plugs*

Neoplasia
- Bladder
- Urethra

Prostatomegaly*

Urethral stricture

Uroliths*
- Bladder neck
- Urethra

Small bladder

Anuria

Congenital hypoplasia

Ectopic ureters

Feline lower urinary tract disease

Non-distensible bladder
- Diffuse bladder wall neoplasia
  - Severe cystitis, e.g.
  - Calculi*
  - Infection*
  - Trauma*

Recent voiding*

Ruptured bladder

Ruptured ureters

Decreased opacity

Emphysematous cystitis

Iatrogenic

Increased opacity

Chronic cystitis*

Foreign body
Neoplasia
Radiopaque calculi*
- Oxalate
- Silica
- Struvite
Superimposition of other organs

Thickening of the bladder wall (contrast cystography)
Chronic cystitis*
Chronic outflow obstruction
Polyps
Small bladder*

Neoplasia
Adenocarcinoma
Leiomyoma
Leiomyosarcoma
Metastatic neoplasia
Rhabdomyosarcoma
Squamous cell carcinoma
Transitional cell carcinoma

Non-visualisation
Ascites
Bladder hypoplasia
Bladder rupture
Empty bladder
- Bilateral ectopic ureters
- Cystitis*
- Post voiding*
Lack of abdominal fat
Positioning fault

3.2.7 Urethra

Contrast medium leakage
Hypospadia
Normal
Previous urethrotomy/urethrostomy

Prostatic disease*
Urethral rupture
- Iatrogenic
- Trauma

Displacement
Adjacent neoplasia
Bladder displacement
Prostatic disease*

Filling defects (contrast urethrography)
Air bubbles*
Blood clots
Neoplasia
Uroliths*

Strictures/irregular surface
Neoplasia
Previous surgery
Previous uroliths
Prostatic disease*
Urethritis*

3.2.8 Kidneys

Dilatation of the renal pelvis (contrast radiography)
Chronic pyelonephritis
Diuresis
Ectopic ureter
Nephrolithiasis or ureterolithiasis
Renal neoplasia

Hydronephrosis
Extrinsic mass
Neoplasia
- Bladder
- Prostate
- Trigone
Paraureteral pseudocyst
Ureteral blood clot

Ureteral inflammation
Ureteral stricture
Ureterolith

Renal pelvic blood clot
Coagulopathy
Iatrogenic (post biopsy)
Idiopathic renal haemorrhage
Neoplasia
Trauma

Enlargement

Irregular outline
Abscess
Cyst
Granuloma
Haematoma
Infarction
Neoplasia
- Adenoma
- Anaplastic sarcoma
- Cystadenocarcinoma
- Haemangioma/haemangiosarcoma
- Metastatic neoplasia
- Nephroblastoma
- Papilloma
- Renal cell carcinoma
- Transitional cell carcinoma
Polycystic kidney disease

Smooth outline
Acute pyelonephritis
Acute kidney injury *q.v.*
Amyloidosis
Compensatory renal hypertrophy
Congenital conditions
- Ectopic ureter
- Ureterocoele
Feline infectious peritonitis* (C)
Hydronephrosis
- Extrinsic mass

- Neoplasia, e.g.
  - Bladder
  - Prostate
  - Trigone
- Paraureteral pseudocyst
- Ureteral blood clot
- Ureteral inflammation
- Ureterolith
- Ureteral stricture

Neoplasia, e.g.
- Lymphoma*

Nephritis*
Perirenal pseudocysts
Portosystemic shunts
Subcapsular abscess
Subcapsular haematoma

Increased radiopacity

Nephroliths

Artefact

Superimposition

Dystrophic mineralisation

Abscess
Granuloma
Haematoma
Neoplasia
Osseous metaplasia

Nephrocalcinosis

Chronic kidney disease* *q.v.*
Ethylene glycol toxicity
Hyperadrenocorticism
Hypercalcaemia *q.v.*
Nephrotoxic drugs
Renal telangiectasia

Non-visualisation

Artefact/technical factors
Nephrectomy

Obscured by gastrointestinal tract contents*
Reduced intra-abdominal contrast* *q.v.*
Retroperitoneal effusion
- Haemorrhage
- Urine
Unilateral renal agenesis
Very small kidneys

Small kidneys

Chronic glomerulonephritis
Chronic interstitial nephritis*
Chronic pyelonephritis

3.2.9   Loss of intra-abdominal contrast

Artefact

Ultrasound gel on coat*
Wet hair coat*

Ascites/peritoneal fluid

Bile

Ruptured biliary tract
- Cholelithiasis
- Neoplasia
- Post surgery, e.g.
  - Cholecystectomy
- Severe cholecystitis
- Trauma

Blood

Angiostrongylus vasorum
Coagulopathy *q.v.*
Neoplasia*, e.g.
- Haemangiosarcoma
Trauma

Chyle

Lymphangiectasia

Ruptured cisterna chyli
- Neoplasia
- Trauma

Exudate

Feline infectious peritonitis* (C)
Septic peritonitis, e.g.
- Iatrogenic/nosocomial
- Neoplasia*
- Pancreatitis*
- Penetrating wound
- Ruptured viscus
  - Neoplasia*
  - Post surgery, e.g.
  - Enterotomy wound dehiscence*
  - Trauma*

Transudate/modified transudate, e.g.

Cardiac tamponade
Caudal vena caval obstruction
Hepatic disease
- Cholangiohepatitis*
- Chronic hepatitis*
- Cirrhosis*
- Fibrosis*
Hypoalbuminaemia* *q.v.*
Neoplasia
Portal hypertension
Right-sided heart failure*

Urine

Lower urinary tract rupture
- Bladder
- Ureter
- Urethra

Diffuse peritoneal neoplasia
Lack of abdominal fat

Emaciation*
Immaturity*

Peritonitis

Irritant
Bile
Urine

Miscellaneous
Neoplasia
Pancreatitis*

Septic
Bile leakage
Gastrointestinal tract leakage
- Devitalisation
  - Foreign body*
  - Gastric dilatation/volvulus*
  - Intestinal volvulus
  - Intussusception
- Perforation
  - Enterotomy wound dehiscence*
  - Gastroduodenal ulceration
  - Penetrating wound
Hepatic abscess
Ruptured prostatic abscess
Ruptured uterus
Septicaemia*
Splenic abscesses
Urinary tract disruption

Viral
Feline infectious peritonitis* (C)

3.2.10 Prostate

Displacement
Abdominal weakness
Full bladder*
Perineal hernia*
Prostatomegaly*

Enlargement
Benign prostatic hyperplasia*
Paraprostatic cysts

Prostatic cysts
Prostatic neoplasia
Prostatitis*
Testicular neoplasia*

3.2.11 Uterus

Enlargement
Haemometra
Hydrometra
Mucometra
Neoplasia
Post partum*
Pregnancy*
Pyometra*
Torsion

3.2.12 Abdominal masses

Cranial abdomen
Adrenal mass
Hepatomegaly/hepatic mass* *q.v.*
Pancreatic mass
Stomach distension/mass*

Mid abdomen
Cryptorchidism*
Mesenteric lymphadenopathy*
Ovarian masses*
Pancreatic enlargement
Renomegaly/renal mass* *q.v.*
Small intestine
- Foreign body*
- Neoplasia*
- Obstruction*
Splenomegaly/splenic mass* *q.v.*

Caudal abdomen
Distended urinary bladder* *q.v.*

Enlarged uterus* *q.v.*
Large intestine
- Foreign body*
- Neoplasia
- Obstruction*
Lymphadenopathy
Prostatomegaly*

3.2.13 Abdominal calcification/mineral density

Abdominal fat
Idiopathic
Pansteatitis

Adrenal glands
Idiopathic
Neoplasia

Arteries
Arteriosclerosis

Gastrointestinal tract
Foreign bodies and ingesta*
Iatrogenic
- Contrast media
- Medication
Uraemic gastritis* *q.v.*

Genital tract
Chronic prostatitis*
Cryptorchidism*
Neoplasia
Ovarian neoplasia
Ovarian or prostatic cyst*
Pregnancy*

Liver
Abscess
Cholelithiasis

Chronic cholecystitis*
Chronic hepatopathy*
Cyst
Granuloma
Haematoma
Neoplasia
Nodular hyperplasia*

Lymph nodes

Inflammation*
Neoplasia*

Miscellaneous

Calcinosis cutis
Chronic hygroma
Foreign body*
Mammary gland neoplasia*
Myositis ossificans

Pancreas

Chronic pancreatitis*
Fat necrosis
Neoplasia
Pancreatic pseudocyst

Spleen

Abscess
Haematoma*
Histoplasmosis

Urinary tract

Chronic inflammation*
Neoplasia
Nephrocalcinosis
- Chronic kidney disease* *q.v.*
- Hyperadrenocorticism
- Hypercalcaemia* *q.v.*
- Nephrotoxic drugs *q.v.*
Urolithiasis*

3.3 Skeletal radiography

3.3.1 Fractures

Congenital/inherited weakness, e.g.
Incomplete ossification of the humeral condyle

Iatrogenic
Bone biopsy
Complication of orthopaedic surgery

Pathological
Bone cyst
Osteopenia *q.v.*

Neoplasia
Chondrosarcoma
Fibrosarcoma
Haemangiosarcoma
Metastatic neoplasia
Multilobular osteochondrosarcoma
Multiple myeloma
Osteosarcoma*

Osteomyelitis
Bacterial*
Fungal
Protozoal, e.g.
• Leishmaniasis

Traumatic*

3.3.2 Altered shape of the long bones

Abnormally straight
Premature closure of growth plate

Angulation
Fractures*

Bowing

Asymmetric growth plate bridging
Iatrogenic, e.g.
Plating
Metaphyseal osteopathy
Chondrodysplasia
Chondrodystrophy
• May be normal breed variation*
Congenital hypothyroidism
Rickets
Tension
• Quadriceps contracture
• Shortening of the ulna

Irregular margination

Calcifying tendinopathy
Bone cyst
• Enchondromatosis
Metaphyseal osteopathy
Neoplasia
• Chondrosarcoma
• Multiple cartilaginous exostoses
• Osteosarcoma*
Periosteal remodelling *q.v.*

3.3.3 Dwarfism

Disproportionate

Chondrodysplasia
Hypervitaminosis A
Hypothyroidism
Mucolipidosis type II
Mucopolysaccharidosis
Rickets

Proportionate

Hypothyroidism
Pituitary dwarfism

3.3.4 Delayed ossification/growth plate closure

Chondrodysplasia
Copper deficiency
Early neutering
Hypervitaminosis D
Hypothyroidism (D)
Mucopolysaccharidosis
Pituitary dwarfism

3.3.5 Increased radiopacity

Artefact
Bone infarcts
Folding fractures*
Growth arrest lines
Lead poisoning
Metaphyseal osteopathy
Neoplasia
Panosteitis
Skeletal immaturity* (metaphyseal condensation)

Osteomyelitis
Bacterial*
Fungal
Protozoal, e.g.
• Leishmaniasis

Osteopetrosis
Acquired
• Chronic excess dietary intake of calcium
• Chronic hypervitaminosis D
• Feline leukaemia virus* (C)
• Idiopathic
• Myelofibrosis
Congenital

3.3.6 Periosteal reactions

Craniomandibular osteopathy
Hip dysplasia*
Hypertrophic osteopathy
Hypervitaminosis A
Metaphyseal osteopathy
Mucopolysaccharidosis
Neoplasia
Panosteitis
Trauma*

Infection
Bacterial*
Fungal
Protozoal
- Hepatozoonosis
- Leishmaniasis
Tuberculosis

3.3.7 Bony masses

Neoplasia

Benign
Chondroma
Endochondroma
Monostotic osteochondroma
Multiple osteochondroma (C)
Osteoma
Polyostotic osteochondroma/multiple cartilaginous exostoses

Malignant
Locally invasive soft tissue
Malignant melanoma of the digit
Soft tissue sarcomas
Squamous cell carcinoma of the digit
Primary bone
- Chondrosarcoma
- Fibrosarcoma

- Giant cell tumour
- Haemangiosarcoma
- Liposarcoma
- Lymphoma
- Multiple myeloma
- Multilobular osteochondrosarcoma
- Osteosarcoma
- Parosteal osteosarcoma
- Plasma cell tumour
- Undifferentiated sarcoma

Tumours which metastasise to bone
- Mammary carcinoma
- Prostatic carcinoma
- Pulmonary carcinoma
- Sarcomas of the rib/chest wall

Miscellaneous
Craniomandibular osteopathy
Enthesopathies

Proliferative joint disease
Disseminated skeletal hyperostosis
Feline periosteal proliferative polyarthropathy (C)
Hypervitaminosis A
Osteoarthritis*

Trauma
Callus*
Hypertrophic non-union
Periosteal reaction

3.3.8   Osteopenia

Artefact

Disuse
Fracture*
Lameness*
Paralysis

Iatrogenic

Chronic anticonvulsant therapy, e.g.
Phenobarbitone
Phenytoin
Primidone
Chronic glucocorticoid administration
Stress protection from plating/casting

Metabolic/endocrine/systemic

Diabetes mellitus*
Hyperadrenocorticism
Hyperthyroidism* (C)
Lactation*
Mucopolysaccharidosis
Pregnancy*
Primary hyperparathyroidism
Renal secondary hyperparathyroidism*

Miscellaneous

Ageing changes
Osteogenesis imperfecta
Panosteitis

Neoplasia

Multiple myeloma
Pseudohyperparathyroidism (see succeeding text)

Nutrition

Chronic protein malnutrition
Hypervitaminosis A
Hyper-/hypovitaminosis D
Nutritional secondary hyperparathyroidism
Pseudohyperparathyroidism
- Adenocarcinoma of the apocrine glands of anal sacs
- Gastric squamous cell carcinoma
- Lymphoma*
- Mammary adenocarcinoma
- Multiple myeloma

- Testicular interstitial cell tumour
- Thyroid adenocarcinoma

Rickets

Toxins

Lead poisoning

3.3.9 Osteolysis

Avascular necrosis of the femoral head* (D)
Bone cysts
Feline femoral metaphyseal osteopathy (C)
Fibro-osseous dysplasia
Fibrous dysplasia
Infarct
Intraosseous epidermoid cysts
Metaphyseal osteopathy
Pressure atrophy
Retained cartilaginous core
Trauma*

Infection

Bacterial

- Bone abscess
- Iatrogenic, e.g. around surgical implants*
- Osteomyelitis*
- Sequestrum

Fungal

Protozoal

- Leishmaniasis

Neoplasia

Enchondroma
Malignant soft tissue tumour
Metastatic tumour
Multiple myeloma
Osteochondroma/multiple cartilaginous exostoses
Osteoclastoma

3.3.10 Mixed osteolytic/osteogenic lesions

Infection

Bacterial
Osteomyelitis*
Sequestrum

Fungal
Aspergillosis
Blastomycosis
Coccidioidomycosis
Cryptococcosis
Histoplasmosis

Protozoal
Leishmaniasis

Neoplasia

Chondrosarcoma
Fibrosarcoma
Haemangiosarcoma
Liposarcoma
Malignant soft tissue tumour*
Metastatic*
Osteosarcoma*

3.3.11 Joint changes

Joint space – increased size

Degenerative joint disease
Intra-articular soft tissue mass
Joint effusion*
Juvenile animal
Positioning artefact/traction
Subluxation

Epiphyseal dysplasia
Chondrodysplasia
Congenital hypothyroidism

Mucopolysaccharidosis
Pituitary dwarfism

Subchondral osteolysis
Neoplasia
Osteochondrosis
Rheumatoid arthritis
Septic arthritis*

Joint space – reduced size
Degenerative joint disease*
Erosive rheumatoid arthritis
Erosive septic arthritis
Periarticular fibrosis
Positioning artefact*

Mixed osteolytic/proliferative joint disease
Avascular necrosis of the femoral head* (D)
Feline periosteal proliferative
polyarthropathy (C)
Feline tuberculosis (C)
Leishmaniasis
Neoplasia
Non-infectious erosive polyarthritis
Osteochondromatosis
Periosteal proliferative polyarthritis
Repeated haemarthroses
Rheumatoid arthritis
Septic arthritis*
Villonodular synovitis

Osteolytic joint disease
Avascular necrosis of the femoral head* (D)
Chronic haemarthrosis
Epiphyseal dysplasia causing apparent osteolysis
Incomplete ossification in juveniles
Osteochondrosis
Osteopenia *q.v.*

Rheumatoid arthritis
Subchondral cysts
Villous nodular synovitis

Infection
Feline tuberculosis (C)
Leishmaniasis
Mycoplasmosis
Septic arthritis*

Neoplasia
Metastatic digital carcinoma
Synovial sarcoma
Other soft tissue neoplasia

Proliferative joint disease
Disseminated idiopathic skeletal
hyperostosis
Enthesopathies
Hypervitaminosis A
Mucopolysaccharidosis
Systemic lupus erythematosus

Neoplasia
Osteoma
Osteosarcoma*
Synovial osteochondroma

Osteoarthritis
Ageing*
Angular limb deformities
Chondrodysplasia
Elbow dysplasia*
Hip dysplasia*
Post articular fractures*
Post surgery*
Other chronic joint stresses
Repeated haemarthroses
Soft tissue damage, e.g.
• Ruptured cranial cruciate ligament*

Soft tissue swelling – joint effusion

Haemarthrosis
Ligament injury
Osteoarthrosis
Osteochondrosis
Shar Pei fever (D)
Soft tissue callus
Synovial cyst
Trauma*
Villonodular synovitis

Arthritis

Iatrogenic
- Drugs, e.g.
  - Sulphonamides
- Vaccine reactions

Idiopathic polyarthritis
Immune-mediated disease
- Arthritis of the Akita (D)
- Gastrointestinal disease associated
- Idiopathic
- Neoplasia associated
- Polyarteritis nodosa
- Polyarthritis/meningitis
- Polyarthritis/polymyositis
- Systemic lupus erythematosus
- Vaccine reaction

Infection
- Borreliosis
- Ehrlichiosis
- Sepsis (bacterial)*

Periarticular swelling

Abscess*
Cellulitis*
Haematoma
Neoplasia
Oedema*

3.4 Radiography of the head and neck

3.4.1 Increased radiopacity/bony proliferation of the maxilla

Acromegaly
Healing/healed fracture*
Neoplasia
Osteomyelitis*

3.4.2 Decreased radiopacity of the maxilla

Granuloma
Nasolacrimal duct cysts

Hyperparathyroidism

Nutritional secondary
Primary
Renal secondary*

Neoplasia

Fibrosarcoma
Local extension of tumour, e.g.
• From nasal cavity*
Malignant melanoma
Osteosarcoma*
Squamous cell carcinoma

Odontogenic cysts

Adamantinoma
Ameloblastoma
Complex odontoma
Dentigerous cyst

Periodontal disease*

3.4.3　Increased radiopacity/bony proliferation of the mandible

Acromegaly
Canine leukocyte adhesion deficiency (D)
Craniomandibular osteopathy
Healing/healed fracture*
Neoplasia
Osteomyelitis*

3.4.4　Decreased radiopacity of the mandible

Granuloma
Periodontal disease

Hyperparathyroidism

Nutritional secondary
Primary
Renal secondary*

Neoplasia

Fibrosarcoma
Malignant melanoma
Osteosarcoma*
Squamous cell carcinoma

Odontogenic cysts

Adamantinoma
Ameloblastoma
Complex odontoma
Dentigerous cyst

3.4.5　Increased radiopacity of the tympanic bulla

Abnormal contents

Cholesteatoma
Granuloma

Neoplasia
Otitis media*
Polyp*

Artefact
Positioning

Thickening of the bulla wall
Canine leukocyte adhesion deficiency (D)
Craniomandibular osteopathy
Neoplasia
Otitis media*
Polyp*

3.4.6 Decreased radiopacity of the nasal cavity

Artefact
Turbinate destruction
Aspergillosis
Congenital defect of the hard palate
Chronic rhinitis, e.g. viral
Destruction of the palatine or maxillary bone, e.g.
  • Neoplasia*
Foreign body*
Previous rhinotomy

3.4.7 Increased radiopacity of the nasal cavity

Artefact

Epistaxis *q.v.*

Miscellaneous
Foreign body
Hyperparathyroidism
Kartagener's syndrome

Polyp
Primary ciliary dyskinesia

Neoplasia

Nasal cavity*
Adenocarcinoma*
Chondrosarcoma
Esthesioneuroblastoma
Fibrosarcoma
Haemangiosarcoma
Histiocytoma
Leiomyosarcoma
Liposarcoma
Lymphoma*
Malignant fibrous histiocytoma
Malignant melanoma
Malignant nerve sheath tumour
Mast cell tumour
Myxosarcoma
Neuroendocrine tumours
Osteosarcoma
Paranasal meningioma
Rhabdomyosarcoma
Squamous cell carcinoma*
Transitional cell carcinoma
Transmissible venereal tumour
Undifferentiated carcinomas*
Undifferentiated sarcoma

Nasal planum
Cutaneous lymphoma
Fibroma
Fibrosarcoma
Haemangioma
Mast cell tumour*
Melanoma
Squamous cell carcinoma

Rhinitis* *q.v.*

3.4.8 Increased radiopacity of the frontal sinuses

Miscellaneous
Canine leukocyte adhesion deficiency (D)
Craniomandibular osteopathy

Neoplasia
Carcinoma*
Local extension, e.g.
- Nasal tumour*
Osteoma
Osteosarcoma

Obstruction of drainage
Neoplasia*
Trauma*

Sinusitis
Allergic*
Bacterial*
Fungal
Kartagener's syndrome
Viral*

3.4.9 Increased radiopacity of the pharynx

Foreign body*
Mineralisation of laryngeal cartilages
Nasopharyngeal stenosis
Obesity*
Pharyngeal paralysis
Salivary calculi

Pharyngeal soft tissue mass
Abscess*
Granuloma
Nasopharyngeal polyp*
Neoplasia

- Carcinoma
- Lymphoma

Retropharyngeal mass

Abscess*
Enlarged lymph nodes*
Neoplasia, e.g.
- Lymphoma*

Soft palate thickening

Brachycephalic obstructive airway syndrome* (D)
Mass
- Cyst
- Granuloma
- Neoplasia

3.4.10   Thickening of the soft tissues of the head and neck

Diffuse

Acromegaly
Cellulitis*
Cranial vena cava syndrome
Neoplasia*
Obesity*
Oedema*

Focal

Abscess*
Cyst*
Foreign body*
Granuloma
Haematoma*
Iatrogenic, e.g.
- Subcutaneous fluid administration*
Neoplasia*

3.4.11 Decreased radiopacity of the soft tissues of the head and neck

Fat
Lipoma*
Obesity*

Gas
Abscess*
Perforation
- Oesophagus
- Pharynx
- Skin
- Trachea
Pneumomediastinum

3.4.12 Increased radiopacity of the soft tissues of the head and neck

Artefact

Calcification
Calcinosis circumscripta
Calcinosis cutis

Calcification of
Abscess
Granuloma
Haematoma
Tumour

Foreign body*

Iatrogenic
Barium
Microchip

Neoplasia

3.5 Radiography of the spine

3.5.1 Normal and congenital variation in vertebral shape and size

Congenital variation

Abnormal dorsal angulation of the
dens of C2

Agenesis/incomplete development
of the dens of C2

Anomalous development of a transverse process
of a lumbar vertebra

Block vertebrae

Butterfly vertebrae

Cervical vertebral malformation–malarticulation syndrome
(wobbler syndrome)* (D)

Chondrodystrophic dwarfism

Congenital metabolic disease

- Congenital hypothyroidism
- Pituitary dwarfism

Fused dorsal spinal processes

Hemivertebrae

Mucopolysaccharidosis

Narrowed vertebral canal

- Cervical vertebral malformation–malarticulation syndrome
  (wobbler syndrome) (D)
- Congenital lumbosacral stenosis
- Secondary to hemivertebrae
  or block vertebrae
- Thoracic stenosis

Occipital dysplasia

Perocormus

Sacrococcygeal dysgenesis

Scoliosis

Shortened dens of C2

Spina bifida

Spinal stenosis

Transitional vertebrae

Normal variation

C7 may be shorter than adjacent vertebrae.
L7 may be shorter than adjacent vertebrae.
Ventral L3 and L4 may be poorly defined.

3.5.2 Acquired variation in vertebral shape and size

Altered vertebral shape

Hyperparathyroidism
- Nutritional secondary
- Primary
- Renal secondary*

Hypervitaminosis A
Mucopolysaccharidosis
Spondylosis deformans
Trauma
- Fracture*

Neoplasia

Chondrosarcoma
Fibrosarcoma
Haemangiosarcoma
Metastatic neoplasia*
- Haemangiosarcoma
- Lymphosarcoma
- Prostatic carcinoma

Multiple cartilaginous exostoses
Multiple myeloma
Osteochondroma
Osteosarcoma*

Decreased vertebral size

Discospondylitis
Fracture*
Intervertebral disc herniation* (D)
Mucopolysaccharidosis
Nutritional secondary hyperparathyroidism

Increased vertebral size

Baastrup's disease
Bone cyst

Callus formation secondary to trauma/pathological fracture
Disseminated idiopathic skeletal hyperostosis
Hypervitaminosis A
Mucopolysaccharidosis

Neoplasia

Chondrosarcoma
Fibrosarcoma
Haemangiosarcoma
Metastatic neoplasia*, e.g.
- Haemangiosarcoma
- Lymphosarcoma
- Prostatic carcinoma

Multiple cartilaginous exostoses
Osteochondroma
Osteosarcoma*

Spondylitis

Bacterial, e.g.
- Foreign body*
- Haematogenous
- Puncture wound

Fungal, e.g.
- Actinomycosis
- Aspergillosis
- Coccidioidomycosis

Parasitic, e.g.
- *Spirocerca lupi*

Protozoal, e.g.
- Hepatozoonosis

Spondylosis deformans

Cervical vertebral malformation–malarticulation syndrome
(wobbler syndrome)* (D)
Chronic disc disease* (D)
Degeneration of annulus fibrosis
Discospondylitis
Hemivertebrae
Post surgery
Trauma*

Vertebral canal changes

Widened
Arachnoid cyst
Syringohydromyelia
Tumour

Narrowed
Adjacent bone pathology, e.g.
Callus
Cervical vertebral malformation–malarticulation syndrome
(wobbler syndrome)* (D)
Lumbosacral stenosis

3.5.3 Changes in vertebral radiopacity

Focal or multifocal decrease in radiopacity

Discospondylitis
Osteomyelitis*
Vertebral physitis

Neoplasia
Chondrosarcoma
Fibrosarcoma
Haemangiosarcoma
Metastatic neoplasia
Multiple myeloma
Osteochondroma
Osteosarcoma*

Focal or multifocal increase in radiopacity

Neoplasia
Chondrosarcoma
Fibrosarcoma
Haemangiosarcoma
Metastatic neoplasia*, e.g.
- Haemangiosarcoma
- Lymphoma
- Prostatic carcinoma

Osteochondroma
Osteosarcoma*

Generalised decrease in radiopacity
Disuse atrophy
Hyperadrenocorticism
Hyperparathyroidism
- Nutritional secondary
- Primary
- Pseudohyperparathyroidism*
- Renal secondary*
Hyperthyroidism* (C)
Hypothyroidism* (D)
Osteogenesis imperfecta
Senile osteoporosis

Generalised increase in radiopacity
Osteopetrosis

3.5.4   Abnormalities in the intervertebral space

Disc space – decreased size
Adjacent hemivertebra
Adjacent neoplasia
Artefact
- Divergence of X-ray beam at periphery of radiograph
- Positioning artefact
Cervical vertebral malformation–malarticulation syndrome
(wobbler syndrome)* (D)
Degenerative canine lumbosacral stenosis
Discospondylitis
Hansen type I disc extrusion* (D)
Hansen type II disc protrusion* (D)
Post surgery
Spondylosis deformans*
Subluxation
Within block vertebra

Disc space – widened
Normal variation
Adjacent to hemivertebra
Artefact (traction)
End-plate erosion
- Discospondylitis
- Neoplasia
Mucopolysaccharidosis
Trauma
- Luxation
- Subluxation

Increased radiopacity of disc space
Artefact
Superimposition of normal
bone/soft tissue
Incidental mineralisation
Intervertebral disc disease* (D)

Irregular margination of disc space
Ageing in cats
Degenerative intervertebral disc disease
Discospondylitis
Mucopolysaccharidosis
Nutritional secondary hyperparathyroidism
Spondylosis deformans*

3.5.5 Contrast radiography of the spine (myelography)

Artefact/technical factors
Contrast medium in soft tissues outside
the vertebral canal
Contrast medium in the spinal parenchyma
Epidural leakage
Injection of contrast into the central canal
Injection of gas into the subarachnoid space
Subdural injection

Extradural lesions

Congenital abnormalities
Foreign body
Neoplasia

Degenerative

Hansen type I disc extrusion* (D)
Hansen type II disc protrusion* (D)
Hansen type III disc high-velocity low-volume extrusion
Hypertrophied ligamentum flavum
Arachnoid cysts

Inflammatory

Abscess
Granuloma

Trauma

Fracture*
Luxation*

Vascular

Haematoma
Haemorrhage

Intradural/extramedullary

Degenerative

Disc disease

Idiopathic

Intra-arachnoid cyst

Inflammatory

Subdural granuloma

Neoplasia

Lymphoma
Meningioma
Nerve root tumour
Nerve sheath tumour

Vascular

Subarachnoid haematoma
Subarachnoid haemorrhage

Intramedullary

Congenital
Syringohydromyelia* (D)

Degenerative
Disc disease* (D)

Inflammatory
Granulomatous meningoencephalomyelitis

Neoplastic
Ependymoma
Glioma
Lymphoma
Metastatic tumours

Traumatic
Cord swelling
- Concussion
- Disc extrusion

Vascular
Ischaemic myelopathy*
Myelomalacia secondary to infarction

Contrast column splitting
Lateralised extradural compression(s)
Midline extradural compression

3.6 Thoracic ultrasonography

3.6.1 Pleural effusion

(See Section 3.1.13 for full listings)
Bile pleuritis
Blood
Chyle
Exudate
Transudate/modified transudate

3.6.2 Mediastinal masses

Granuloma
Idiopathic mediastinal cysts
Neoplasia
- Lymphoma*
- Mast cell tumour
- Melanoma
- Thymoma*
- Thyroid carcinoma
Reactive lymphadenopathy*
Thymic branchial cysts

3.6.3 Pericardial effusion

Secondary to cardiomyopathy (C)*

Haemorrhagic
Coagulopathy *q.v.*
Left atrial rupture

Idiopathic*(D)
Neoplastic*
Haemangiosarcoma
Heart base tumours
- Chemodectoma
- Metastatic parathyroid tumour
- Metastatic thyroid tumour
- Other metastatic tumours*
- Nonchromaffin paraganglioma
Lymphoma
Mesothelioma

Pericarditis
Bacterial
Bite wounds
Extension of pulmonary infection

Foreign bodies
Oesophageal perforation
Fungal
Uraemic
Viral
- Feline infectious peritonitis* (C)

3.6.4 Altered chamber dimensions

LEFT HEART

Left atrial enlargement
Chronic bradycardia
Dilated cardiomyopathy*
Hyperthyroidism* (C)
Hypertrophic cardiomyopathy* (C)
Left-to-right shunt
Mitral dysplasia
Myxomatous degeneration of the mitral valve* (D)
Primary atrial disease
Restrictive cardiomyopathy (C)

Left ventricle

Dilatation
Anaemia
Arteriovenous fistula
Chronic bradycardia *q.v.*
Chronic tachyarrhythmia *q.v.*
Dilated cardiomyopathy
- Drugs/toxins, e.g.
  - Doxorubicin
- Idiopathic*
- Parvovirus
- Taurine deficiency
High-output states
- Anaemia* *q.v.*
- Hyperthyroidism* (C)
Myocarditis
Volume overload

- Aortic insufficiency
- Left-to-right shunts
  - Arteriovenous fistulas
  - Atrial septal defects
  - Patent ductus arteriosus
  - Ventricular septal defects
- Mitral regurgitation, e.g.
  - Mitral dysplasia
  - Myxomatous degeneration of the mitral valve* (D)

Hypertrophy
Cardiomyopathy
Hypertrophic* (C)
Coarctation of the aorta
Endomyocardial fibrosis
Hyperthyroidism* (C)
Infiltrative cardiac disease, e.g.
- Lymphoma
Pressure overload
- Aortic/subaortic stenosis
- Systemic arterial hypertension*
Pseudohypertrophy from volume depletion*

Reduction
Hypovolaemia *q.v.**

Wall thinning
Aneurysm
Dilated cardiomyopathy*
Infarction
Prior myocarditis

RIGHT HEART

Right atrial enlargement
Anaemia *q.v.*
Arteriovenous fistula
Atrial septal defect
Chronic bradycardia
Cor pulmonale
Dilated cardiomyopathy*
Heartworm disease

Hyperthyroidism* (C)
Hypertrophic cardiomyopathy* (C)
Myxomatous degeneration of the tricuspid
valve* (D)
Primary atrial myocardial diseases
Pulmonary hypertension
Restrictive cardiomyopathy (C)
Right-to-left shunts
Tricuspid dysplasia
Tricuspid stenosis/atresia

Right ventricle

Dilatation
Right ventricular volume overload
- Atrial septal defects
- Cardiomyopathy
  - Dilated cardiomyopathy* (D)
  - Hypertrophic cardiomyopathy* (C)
  - Restrictive cardiomyopathy (C)
- Pulmonic insufficiency
- Tricuspid insufficiency
  - Myxomatous degeneration of the
    tricuspid valve* (D)
  - Tricuspid dysplasia

Hypertrophy
Hypertrophic cardiomyopathy* (C)
Pressure overload
- Cor pulmonale
- Heartworm disease
- Large ventricular septal defect
- Pulmonary hypertension
- Pulmonary thromboembolism
- Pulmonic stenosis
- Tetralogy of Fallot
Restrictive cardiomyopathy (C)

Reduction
Cardiac tamponade
Hypovolaemia* *q.v.*

3.6.5 Changes in ejection phase indices of left ventricular performance (fractional shortening, FS%; ejection fraction, EF)

Apparently reduced performance (decreased FS%, decreased EF)

Decreased preload, e.g.
Hypovolaemia* *q.v.*

Increased afterload, e.g.
Aortic stenosis
Systemic arterial hypertension* *q.v.*

Reduced systolic function
Canine X-linked muscular dystrophy
Chronic valvular heart disease* (D)
Dilated cardiomyopathy*

Apparently increased performance (increased FS%, increased EF)

Decreased afterload, e.g.
Hypotension
Mitral valve regurgitation*

Increased preload, e.g.
Iatrogenic fluid overload*

Myocardial disease, e.g.
Hypertrophic cardiomyopathy* (C)

3.7 Abdominal ultrasonography

3.7.1 Renal disease

Diffuse abnormalities
Renomegaly *q.v.*
Small kidneys *q.v.*

Increased cortical echogenicity with normal or enhanced corticomedullary definition
End-stage renal disease* *q.v.*

Ethylene glycol toxicity
Fat in the cortex*
Feline infectious peritonitis* (C)
Glomerulonephritis
Interstitial nephritis*
Nephrocalcinosis
Lymphoma
Squamous cell carcinoma

Medullary rim sign
May be normal*
Chronic interstitial nephritis*
Ethylene glycol toxicity
Feline infectious peritonitis* (C)
Hypercalcaemic nephropathy
Idiopathic acute tubular necrosis
Leptospirosis*

Increased cortical echogenicity with reduced corticomedullary definition
Chronic inflammatory disease*
Congenital renal dysplasia
End-stage kidneys*

Reduced cortical echogenicity
Lymphoma

Focal abnormalities

Anechoic/hypoechoic lesions
Abscess
Acquired cysts secondary to nephropathies
Congenital cysts
Cystadenocarcinoma
Haematoma
Lymphoma
Perirenal pseudocyst
Polycystic kidney disease*
Tumour necrosis

Hyperechoic lesions
Calcified abscess
Calcified cyst wall

Calcified haematoma
  Calculi
  Chronic renal infarcts
  Fibrosis
  Gas
  Granuloma
  Neoplasia
  - Chondrosarcoma
  - Haemangioma
  - Haemangiosarcoma
  - Metastatic thyroid adenocarcinoma
  - Osteosarcoma

Mixed echogenicity lesions
  Abscess
  Acute infarct
  Granuloma
  Haematoma
  Neoplasia
  - Adenocarcinoma
  - Haemangioma
  - Lymphoma

Pelvic dilatation
  Contralateral renal disease/absence
  (mild dilatation)
  Polyuria/diuresis
  Pyelonephritis
  Renal neoplasia

Congenital conditions
  Ectopic ureter
  Ureterocoele

Hydronephrosis
  Extrinsic mass
  Neoplasia
  - Bladder
  - Prostate
  - Trigone
  Paraureteral pseudocyst
  Ureteral blood clot

Ureteral inflammation
Ureteral stricture
Ureterolith

3.7.2 Hepatobiliary disease

Biliary obstruction (see also Jaundice)
Abscess
Biliary calculi
Gastrointestinal disease* *q.v.*
Granuloma
Hepatobiliary disease* *q.v.*
Lymphadenopathy* *q.v.*
Neoplasia*
Pancreatic disease, e.g. pancreatitis*

Diffuse hepatic disease
Hepatomegaly *q.v.**
Microhepatica *q.v.*

Decreased echogenicity
Amyloidosis
Congestion*
Hepatitis*
Leukaemia
Lymphoma*

Increased echogenicity
Chronic hepatitis*
Cirrhosis*
Fatty infiltration
 • Diabetes mellitus*
 • Obesity*
Lymphoma*
Steroid hepatopathy*

Mixed echogenicity
Cirrhosis*
Diffuse neoplasia*
Hepatocutaneous syndrome

Dilatation of the caudal vena cava and hepatic veins
Haematological disorders
Systemic infection*

Obstruction of the caudal vena cava/hepatic veins
Budd–Chiari syndrome
Liver disease* *q.v.*
Neoplasia*
Strictures
Thrombosis
Trauma*

*Right-sided heart failure**
Cardiac tamponade
Dirofilariasis
Myocardial disease
Pulmonary hypertension
Pulmonic stenosis
Tricuspid insufficiency

Focal or multifocal hepatic parenchymal abnormalities
Nodular hyperplasia (D)*

Abscess
Biliary disease*
Chronic glucocorticoid administration
Diabetes mellitus*
Liver lobe torsion
Neoplasia*
Pancreatitis*
Penetrating foreign body

Cysts
Acquired cysts
• Biloma
• Polycystic renal disease*
Congenital cysts

Cyst-like masses
Biliary pseudocyst
Inflammation

Necrosis
Neoplasia*
Trauma

Haematoma
 Coagulopathy *q.v.*
 Trauma*

Hepatic necrosis
 Chemical insult
 Immune mediated*
 Infection*
 Toxin

Neoplasia
 Biliary cystadenoma
 Cholangiocellular adenocarcinoma
 Cholangiocellular adenoma
 Hepatocellular adenocarcinoma*
 Hepatocellular adenoma*
 Lymphoma*
 Metastatic tumours*

Focal/multifocal increased echogenicity of the gall bladder

 Biliary calculi
 Gall bladder mucocoele
 Gall bladder sludge*
 Neoplasia
 Polyps

Gall bladder wall thickening

 Acute hepatitis* *q.v.*
 Cholangiohepatitis*
 Cholecystitis* *q.v.*
 Chronic hepatitis* *q.v.*
 Gall bladder mucocoeles
 Hypoalbuminaemia* *q.v.*
 Neoplasia*
 Right-sided congestive heart failure*
 Sepsis*

3.7.3 Splenic disease

Diffuse splenic disease – splenomegaly

Amyloidosis
Extramedullary haematopoiesis
Immune-mediated disease*
Infarction
Parenchymal necrosis
Portal hypertension
Splenic vein thrombosis

Congestion
Anaesthetic agents*
Haemolytic anaemia*
Portal vein obstruction
Right-sided heart failure*
Torsion of the splenic pedicle
- Gastric dilatation/volvulus
- Isolated
Toxaemia*
Tranquillizers*

Infection
Bacterial*
Fungal

Neoplasia
Lymphoma*
Lymphoproliferative disease
Malignant histiocytosis
Mastocytosis
Myeloproliferative disease

Parasites
Babesiosis
Ehrlichiosis
Haemotropic *Mycoplasma* spp.

Focal or multifocal splenic disease

Abscess
Fat deposits
Nodular hyperplasia

Haematoma
　Abdominal trauma
　Coagulopathy

Infarcts
　Cardiovascular disease*
　Hyperadrenocorticism
　Hypercoagulability
　Inflammatory diseases
　　• Endocarditis
　　• Pancreatitis*
　　• Septicaemia*
　Liver disease* *q.v.*
　Neoplasia*
　　• Fibrosarcoma
　　• Haemangioma
　　• Haemangiosarcoma
　　• Leiomyosarcoma
　　• Lymphoma
　Renal disease* *q.v.*

Neoplasia
　Chondrosarcoma
　Fibrosarcoma
　Fibrous histiocytoma
　Haemangioma*
　Haemangiosarcoma*
　Leiomyosarcoma
　Liposarcoma
　Lymphoma*
　Metastatic tumours*
　Myxosarcoma
　Osteosarcoma
　Rhabdomyosarcoma
　Undifferentiated sarcoma

3.7.4　Pancreatic disease

Focal pancreatic lesions
　Abscess (D)
　Cyst-like structures

- Congenital cysts
- Pseudocysts
- Retention cysts

Neoplasia

Nodular changes

Diffuse enlargement

Pancreatic neoplasia

Pancreatic oedema

Pancreatitis*

3.7.5   Adrenal disease

Adrenomegaly

Unilateral

Adrenal tumour

- Adrenocortical adenocarcinoma*
- Adrenocortical adenoma*
- Blastoma
- Metastatic tumours
- Pheochromocytoma

Bilateral

Adrenal tumours

- Adrenocortical adenocarcinoma*
- Adrenocortical adenoma*
- Metastatic tumours

Drugs

- Trilostane

Hyperplasia

Pituitary-dependent hyperadrenocorticism*

Stressful non-adrenal illness*

3.7.6   Urinary bladder disease

Increased wall thickness

Diffuse

Chronic cystitis*

Emphysematous cystitis
- Clostridial infection
- Diabetes mellitus

Empty bladder*

Fibrosis/calcification of the bladder wall

Focal or multifocal

Mural haematomas
- Coagulopathy *q.v.*
- Iatrogenic
- Infection
- Neoplasia
- Trauma

Neoplasia
- Adenocarcinoma
- Chemodectoma
- Fibroma
- Fibrosarcoma
- Haemangioma
- Haemangiosarcoma
- Leiomyoma
- Leiomyosarcoma
- Lymphoma
- Myxoma
- Rhabdomyosarcoma
- Squamous cell carcinoma
- Transitional cell carcinoma
- Undifferentiated carcinoma

Focal wall defects

Acquired diverticulum
Patent urachus
Urachal diverticulum
Ureterocoele

Intraluminal lesions, e.g.

Blood clots*
Foreign bodies
Gas bubbles
Sediment*
Uroliths*

3.7.7 Gastrointestinal disease

Increased wall thickness

Diffuse

Acute haemorrhagic gastroenteritis*
Colitis* *q.v.*
Gastritis*
- Dietary*
- Infectious*
  - Parvovirus*
- Inflammatory*
- Uraemic* *q.v.*

Inflammatory bowel disease*
Neoplasia
- Lymphoma*

Focal/multifocal

Benign adenomatous polyps
Chronic hypertrophic gastropathy
Congenital hypertrophic pyloric stenosis
Inflammatory bowel disease*
Intussusception (apparent)
Neoplasia
- Adenocarcinoma
- Adenoma
- Carcinoid tumours
- Carcinoma
- Leiomyoma
- Leiomyosarcoma
- Lymphoma
- Neurilemmoma

Decreased intestinal motility (ileus)

Functional

Abdominal pain*
Acute gastroenteritis*
Amyloidosis
Neurogenic disease
Oedema

Post-operative abdomen*
Vascular disease
Drugs

Mechanical
Adhesions*
Foreign body*
Intussusception
Localised inflammation*
Neoplasia

3.7.8 Ovarian and uterine disease

Ovarian masses
Ovarian stump granuloma

*Cysts**
Follicular
Luteinising

Neoplasia
Adenoma
Adenocarcinoma
Dysgerminoma
Granulosa cell tumour
Luteoma
Teratoma
Thecoma

Uterine enlargement
Haemometra
Hydrometra
Mucometra
Post partum*
Pregnancy*
Pyometra*

Uterine wall thickening

Neoplasia
Adenocarcinoma
Adenoma

Fibroma
Fibrosarcoma
Leiomyoma
Leiomyosarcoma
Lymphoma

3.7.9   Prostatic disease

Prostatic enlargement

Diffuse
    Bacterial prostatitis*
    Benign prostatic hyperplasia*
    Neoplasia
    Squamous metaplasia

Focal lesions
    Abscessation
    Cysts
      • Paraprostatic
      • Prostatic
    Neoplasia
      • Adenocarcinoma
      • Fibroma
      • Leiomyoma
      • Leiomyosarcoma
      • Squamous cell carcinoma
      • Transitional cell carcinoma
      • Undifferentiated carcinoma

3.7.10   Ascites

Bile – ruptured biliary tract

    Neoplasia
    Post surgery, e.g.
      • Cholecystectomy
    Severe cholecystitis*
    Trauma

Blood
Coagulopathy
Neoplasia, e.g.
- Haemangiosarcoma*
Organ or major blood vessel rupture
Thrombosis
Trauma
Vasculitis

Chyle
Congestive heart failure
Feline infectious peritonitis (C)
Lymphangiectasia
Lymphangiosarcoma
Lymphoma
Mesenteric root strangulation
Ruptured cisterna chyli
- Neoplasia
- Trauma
Steatitis

Exudate
Diaphragmatic hernia
Feline infectious peritonitis* (C)
Hepatitis
Neoplasia
Organ torsion
Pancreatitis
Pericardiodiaphragmatic hernia

Septic peritonitis
Abscess
Haematogenous spread
Iatrogenic/nosocomial
Local extension of infection from elsewhere
Migrating foreign body
Neoplasia*
Pancreatitis*
Penetrating wound
Primary

Ruptured viscus, e.g.
- Neoplasia
- Post surgery, e.g.
  - Enterotomy wound dehiscence*
- Pyometra
- Trauma

Steatitis

Transudate/modified transudate

Cardiac tamponade *q.v.*
Caudal vena caval obstruction
Hepatic disease
- Cholangiohepatitis* *q.v.*
- Chronic hepatitis* *q.v.*
- Cirrhosis*
- Fibrosis*
- Portal hypertension

Hypoalbuminaemia* *q.v.*
Inflammation
- Feline infectious peritonitis

Neoplasia*
Portal hypertension
Right-sided heart failure*
Ruptured cyst
Splenic disease

Urine – lower urinary tract rupture

Bladder
Ureter
Urethra

3.8 Ultrasonography of other regions

3.8.1 Testes

Enlargement

Neoplasia*
Orchitis
Torsion

Focal lesions – neoplasia
Interstitial cell tumour*
Seminoma*
Sertoli cell tumour*

3.8.2 Eyes

Intraocular masses
Foreign body*
Inflammation*

*Infection**
Bacteria
Fungi
- Blastomycosis
- Coccidioidomycosis
- Cryptococcosis
- Histoplasmosis
Viral
- Feline infectious peritonitis* (C)

Neoplasia
Ciliary body adenocarcinoma
Ciliary body adenoma
Lymphoma
Medulloepithelioma
Melanoma
Metastatic cancer
Squamous cell carcinoma

*Organised haemorrhage**
Chronic glaucoma
Coagulopathy *q.v.*
Diabetes mellitus*
Hypertension* *q.v.*
Neoplasia
Neovascularisation
Persistent hyaloid artery
Trauma*
Vitreoretinal disease

Point-like and membranous lesions of the vitreous chamber

Asteroid hyalosis
Endophthalmitis
Foreign body
Haemorrhage (see preceding text)
Persistent hyperplastic primary vitreous
Posterior vitreal detachment
Vitreous floaters
Vitreous membrane formation

Retinal detachment *q.v.*

Retrobulbar masses

Abscess/cellulitis*

Extension from nasal cavity
Extension from paranasal sinuses
Extension from tooth root infection*
Extension from zygomatic salivary gland
Foreign body
Haematogenous spread
Oral inflammatory disease
Penetrating wound

Neoplasia

Metastatic tumours
Chondrosarcoma
Haemangiosarcoma
Lacrimal gland tumour
Lymphoma
Meningioma
Nasal adenocarcinoma
Neurofibrosarcoma
Osteosarcoma
Rhabdomyosarcoma
Squamous cell carcinoma
Zygomatic gland tumour
Primary epithelial and mesenchymal tumours

3.8.3 Neck

Enlarged parathyroid gland(s)

Neoplasia
Adenocarcinoma
Adenoma

Hyperplasia
Nutritional secondary hyperparathyroidism
Renal secondary hyperparathyroidism

Enlarged thyroid gland(s)

Miscellaneous
Thyroid cyst
Thyroiditis

Neoplasia
Adenocarcinoma*
Adenoma*

Lymph node enlargement

Inflammation/infection
Abscess*
Inflammation*

Neoplasia
Lymphoma*
Metastatic neoplasia*

Salivary gland enlargement

Salivary cysts
Retention cyst
True cyst
Salivary gland abscess*
Salivary gland neoplasia
Sialadenitis/sialadenosis
Sialocoele*
Sialolithiasis

Neck masses at other sites

Inflammation/infection
  Abscess*
  Cellulitis
  Granuloma

Neoplasia
  Lipoma*
  Metastatic neoplasia
  Primary neoplasia

Miscellaneous
  Arteriovenous malformation
  Cyst*
  Haematoma*

PART 4
LABORATORY FINDINGS

In order to avoid repetition, 'laboratory error' has been omitted from the differential diagnoses in this chapter. However, it should always be borne in mind that factors such as mislabelling or misidentification of samples, errors introduced by the laboratory machinery (especially certain in-house laboratories where quality control is inadequate) and errors due to ageing samples or incorrect collection techniques can all cause apparent abnormalities. Where a test result is unexpectedly abnormal, it should be repeated, preferably by a different method. It is also important to remember that reference intervals are usually based on the values into which 95% of the healthy population would fall, so small changes outside these values may not be significant. Finally, each laboratory establishes its own reference intervals, due to differences in testing methodology and local factors, and thus when comparing results over a course of time, it is best to use the same laboratory.

4.1 Biochemical findings

4.1.1 Albumin

Decreased
Relative (dilutional)

Decreased production
Chronic inflammatory disease*
Hepatic failure* *q.v.*

Differential Diagnosis in Small Animal Medicine, Second Edition.
Alex Gough and Kate Murphy.
© 2015 John Wiley & Sons, Ltd. Published 2015 by John Wiley & Sons, Ltd.

Decreased protein intake
  Malabsorption*
  Maldigestion
  Malnutrition

Increased loss
  Cutaneous lesions, e.g.
  • Burns
  External haemorrhage*, e.g.
  • Coagulopathy *q.v.*
  • Gastrointestinal neoplasia
  • Gastrointestinal ulceration
  • External parasites
  • Trauma
  Protein-losing enteropathy*
  • Acute gastrointestinal infection, e.g. viral
  • Cardiac disease
  • Inflammatory bowel disease
  • Gastrointestinal neoplasia
  • Gastrointestinal parasitism
  • Gastrointestinal ulceration
  • Lymphangiectasia
    ◦ Intestinal inflammation
    ◦ Intestinal neoplasia
    ◦ Lymphangitis
    ◦ Primary/congenital
    ◦ Venous hypertension
    ◦ Protein-losing nephropathy *q.v.*

Sequestration
  Body cavity effusion* *q.v.*

Increased
  Artefact
  • Lipaemia
  Haemoconcentration*
  • Dehydration

4.1.2 Alanine transferase

Decreased (minimal clinical significance)
Chronic liver disease
Normal variation*
Nutritional deficiency
- Vitamin B6
- Zinc

Increased

Artefact
Haemolysis
Lipaemia

Drugs/toxins
Barbiturates
Cimetidine
Colchicine
Cyclophosphamide
Danazol
Diazepam (C)
Glucocorticoids
Griseofulvin
Itraconazole
Ketoconazole
Methimazole
Methotrexate
Metronidazole
Mexiletine
Nandrolone
NSAIDs, e.g.
- Ibuprofen
- Paracetamol
- Phenylbutazone
Oxytetracycline
Phenobarbitone
Phenylbutazone
Phenytoin
Primidone

Procainamide
Salicylates
Tetracycline
Trimethoprim/sulphonamide

Extrahepatic disease
Anoxia
Endocrine disease, e.g.
- Hyperadrenocorticism
- Hyperthyroidism (C)
- Diabetes mellitus

Inflammatory disease, e.g.
- Pancreatitis
- Muscle disease, e.g. muscular dystrophy (D), trauma

Hepatic disease
Cholangiohepatitis* *q.v.*
Cholangitis* *q.v.*
Chronic hepatitis* *q.v.*
Cirrhosis*
Copper storage disease (D)
Feline infectious peritonitis* (C)
Hepatotoxin
Lipidosis
Neoplasia, e.g.
- Hepatocellular adenocarcinoma*
- Lymphoma*

Trauma*

4.1.3 Alkaline phosphatase

Increased
Normal in young growing animals*

Artefact
Haemolysis
Hyperbilirubinaemia
Lipaemia

Drugs/toxins
Aflatoxin
Barbiturates
Cimetidine
Colchicine
Cyclophosphamide
Danazol
Diazepam (C)
Glucocorticoids
Griseofulvin
Itraconazole
Ketoconazole
Methimazole
Methotrexate
Metronidazole
Mexiletine
Nandrolone
NSAIDs, e.g.
- Ibuprofen
- Paracetamol
- Phenylbutazone

Oxytetracycline
Phenobarbitone
Phenoxy acid herbicides
Phenylbutazone
Phenytoin
Primidone
Procainamide
Salicylates
Trimethoprim/sulphonamide

Extrahepatic disease
Bile duct neoplasia
Bone disease, e.g.
- Fracture
- Osteomyelitis

Cholecystitis*
Cholelithiasis
Diabetes mellitus*
Diaphragmatic hernia*

Ehrlichiosis
Gall bladder mucocoele
Hyperadrenocorticism
Hyperthyroidism (C)*
Pancreatic neoplasia
Pancreatitis*
Right-sided congestive heart failure*
Septicaemia*

Hepatic disease

Cholangiohepatitis* *q.v.*
Chronic hepatitis* *q.v.*
Cirrhosis* *q.v.*
Copper storage disease (D)
Feline infectious peritonitis* (C)
Hepatic lipidosis (C)
Hepatic neoplasia*, e.g.
- Haemangiosarcoma
- Hepatocellular carcinoma
- Lymphoma
- Metastatic carcinoma

4.1.4 Ammonia

Decreased (minimal clinical significance)

Drugs
Diphenhydramine
Enemas
Lactulose
Oral antibiotics, e.g.
- Aminoglycosides
- Probiotics

Increased

Artefact
Delay in sample analysis
Fluoride/oxalate anticoagulants
Strenuous exercise

Drugs
   Ammonium salts
   Asparaginase
   Diuretics

Hepatic insufficiency
   Decreased functional hepatic mass, e.g.
   • Diffuse chronic hepatic disease
   Decreased portal blood flow to the liver, e.g.
   • Acquired portosystemic shunt
   • Congenital portosystemic shunt

Miscellaneous
   High-protein diet*
   Intestinal haemorrhage
   Urea cycle disorders
   Selective cobalamin deficiency, e.g. border collie

4.1.5 Amylase

Increased

Drugs/toxins
   Azathioprine
   Carbamate
   Diazoxide
   Frusemide
   Glucocorticoids
   L-Asparaginase
   Metronidazole
   Oestrogens
   Potassium bromide
   Sulphonamides
   Tetracyclines
   Thiazide diuretics

Intestinal disease*

*Pancreatic disease**
   Necrosis
   Neoplasia

Pancreatic duct obstruction
Pancreatitis*

Reduced glomerular filtration q.v.

Pre-renal disease*
Renal disease*
Post-renal disease*

4.1.6 Aspartate aminotransferase

Increased

Artefact

Haemolysis
Lipaemia

Drugs/toxins

Barbiturates
Carbamate
Glucocorticoids
Griseofulvin
Ketoconazole
NSAIDs, e.g.
- Ibuprofen
- Paracetamol
- Phenobarbitone
- Phenylbutazone
- Primidone
- Salicylates

*Haemolysis**

Hepatic disease q.v.*
*Muscle damage**

Exercise
Inflammation
Intramuscular injection
Ischaemia
Necrosis
Neoplasia
Trauma

4.1.7 Bilirubin

Decreased (minimal clinical significance)

Artefact
Prolonged exposure to sunlight
or fluorescent light

Increased (see also Jaundice)

Artefact
Haemolysis
Lipaemia

Drugs/toxins
Barbiturates
Blue-green algae
Glucocorticoids
Glyphosphate
Griseofulvin
Ketoconazole
Metronidazole
Phenobarbitone
Plastic explosives
Primidone
NSAIDs, e.g.
- Ibuprofen
- Paracetamol
- Phenylbutazone
Salicylates

Pre-hepatic
Haemolysis*

Hepatic, e.g.
Diffuse hepatocellular disease
Cholestatic liver disease* *q.v.*

Post-hepatic, e.g.
Biliary obstruction* *q.v.*

Miscellaneous
Bile sludging with dehydration and anorexia (C)
Decreased rate of excretion (functional cholestasis) in sepsis

4.1.8 Bile acids/dynamic bile acid test

Failure to stimulate
Cholestyramine
Delayed gastric emptying
Failure to feed a sufficiently high-fat meal for bile
acid stimulation test
Malabsorption
Rapid intestinal transit time
Normal

Increased
Artefact
Haemolysis
Lipaemia
Decreased bile acid removal from portal blood
Portosystemic shunt
- Acquired
- Congenital
Decreased excretion bile acids
Hepatic disease
Cholestatic disease* *q.v.*
Hepatic parenchymal disease* *q.v.*
Secondary hepatic disease*
Drugs
- Ursodeoxycholic acid

4.1.9 C-reactive protein (D)

Decreased
Severe obesity

Increased
Extreme exercise
Inflammation*, e.g.

Arthritis (including IMPA)
Haemolytic anaemia, pancreatitis, SRMA
Infection, e.g.
   Bordetella
   E. coli
   Ehrlichia
   Leishmania
   Parvovirus
   Pyometra
Neoplasia*, e.g.
Haemangiosarcoma
Leukaemia
Lymphoma
Parturition*
Pregnancy (period of time)
Tissue trauma*

4.1.10 Cholesterol

Decreased

Artefact
   Intravenous dipyrone

Drugs
   Azathioprine
   Oral aminoglycosides

Gastrointestinal
   Hepatic insufficiency* *q.v.*
   Maldigestion/malabsorption* *q.v.*
   Protein-losing enteropathy* *q.v.*

Increased

   Idiopathic hyperlipidaemia
   Postprandial hyperlipidaemia

Artefact
   Hyperbilirubinaemia
   Lipaemia

Drugs
    Corticosteroids
    Phenytoin
    Thiazide diuretics

Breed related
    Hypercholesterolaemia of the briard, rough collie and Shetland
    sheepdog (D)

Secondary hyperlipidaemia
    Cholestatic disease* *q.v.*
    Diabetes mellitus*
    Hyperadrenocorticism
    Hypothyroidism* (D)
    Nephrotic syndrome
    Pancreatic disease
    Protein-losing nephropathy

4.1.11 Creatinine

Decreased
    Poor body condition

Increased
    Increased protein catabolism, e.g. heavily muscled dogs
    Pre-renal azotaemia*
    Renal azotaemia*
    • Acute kidney injury
    • Chronic kidney disease
    Post-renal azotaemia*
    • (See Urea *q.v.*)

4.1.12 Creatine kinase

Mild increase (e.g. 2–3x upper reference interval)
    Intramuscular injections*
    Muscle biopsy
    Muscle damage
    Physical activity*

Prolonged recumbency*
Restraint*

Moderate to marked increase
Anorexia
Convulsions*
Endocrine, e.g.
    Hyperadrenocorticism
    Hypothyroidism (D)
    Hyperthyroidism (C)
Feline lower urinary tract disease
Masticatory myopathy
Muscle damage
Myopathies
    • *Inherited, e.g.*
      Hereditary Labrador retriever myopathy
      Muscular dystrophy
      Myotonia
    • *Inflammatory/infectious, e.g.*
      Immune-mediated polymyositis
      Neosporosis
      Toxoplasmosis
    • *Nutritional, e.g.*
      Selenium deficiency
      Vitamin E deficiency
Neuropathies
Toxins, e.g.
    • Carbamate
    • Lily poisoning
    • Monensin
    • Phenoxy acid herbicides
Thromboembolic disease
Trauma*
Tremors/shivering *q.v.*

4.1.13 Ferritin

Decreased
Iron deficiency disorders *q.v.*
Acute/chronic inflammation

Portosystemic shunts
Young animals

Increased

Cortisol excess (D)
Haemolysis*
Iatrogenic, e.g.
  • Injections, diet
Inflammation*
Liver disease*
Neoplasia*
  • Lymphoma
Repeated blood transfusions

4.1.14   Fibrinogen

Decreased

Artefact
  • Clot
  • Incorrect anticoagulant
Disseminated intravascular coagulation*
Excessive blood loss*
Hereditary fibrinogen deficiency/abnormality
Severe hepatic insufficiency

Increased

Breed related
  • Cavalier King Charles spaniels
Haemoconcentration
Inflammation*
Parturition*
Pregnancy*
Renal disease*

4.1.15   Folate

Decreased

Dietary deficiency
Proximal small intestinal disease*

Increased
Dietary/parenteral supplementation
Exocrine pancreatic insufficiency
Small intestinal bacterial overgrowth*

4.1.16 Fructosamine

Decreased
Hyperthyroidism (C)
Insulin overdosage
Persistent hypoglycaemia *q.v.*, e.g.
- Insulinoma

Increased
Hypothyroidism (D)*
Persistent hyperglycaemia, e.g.
- Diabetes mellitus*

4.1.17 Gamma-glutamyl transferase

Increased

Artefact
Lipaemia

Drugs
Barbiturates
Glucocorticoids
Griseofulvin
Ketoconazole
NSAIDs, e.g.
- Ibuprofen
- Paracetamol
- Phenylbutazone

Phenobarbitone
Primidone
Salicylates

Extrahepatic disease
  Bile duct neoplasia
  Cholecystitis*
  Cholelithiasis
  Diabetes mellitus*
  Diaphragmatic hernia*
  Gall bladder mucocoele
  Hyperadrenocorticism
  Hyperthyroidism (C)*
  Pancreatic neoplasia
  Pancreatitis*
  Right-sided congestive heart failure*
  Septicaemia*

Hepatic disease
  Cholangiohepatitis* *q.v.*
  Chronic hepatitis* *q.v.*
  Cirrhosis* *q.v.*
  Copper storage disease (D)
  Feline infectious peritonitis* (C)
  Hepatic lipidosis (C)
  Hepatic neoplasia*, e.g.
  • Haemangiosarcoma
  • Hepatocellular carcinoma
  • Lymphoma
  • Metastatic carcinoma

4.1.18 Gastrin

Increased
  Antral G-cell hyperplasia
  Atrophic gastritis
  Chronic omeprazole administration
  Gastric outlet obstruction
  Gastrinoma
  Hyperparathyroidism
  Renal disease* *q.v.*
  Short bowel syndrome

4.1.19 Globulins

Decreased

Normal in greyhounds
External haemorrhage, e.g.
- Coagulopathy *q.v.*
- Gastrointestinal neoplasia
- Gastrointestinal ulceration
- Trauma*

Hepatic insufficiency* *q.v.*
Neonate*
Protein-losing enteropathies* *q.v.*

Increased

Polyclonal

Dehydration
Infectious disease
  Bacterial disease*, e.g.
- Bacterial endocarditis
  - Brucellosis
  - Pyoderma*

  Fungal disease, e.g.
- Blastomycosis
  - Coccidioidomycosis
  - Histoplasmosis

  Parasitic disease*, e.g.
- Demodicosis*
  - Dirofilariasis
  - Scabies*

  Protozoal disease
  Rickettsial disease, e.g.
- Ehrlichiosis
  - Viral disease*, e.g.
  - Feline immunodeficiency virus* (C)
  - Feline infectious peritonitis* (C)
  - Feline leukaemia virus* (C)

Immune mediated/inflammatory
  Acute inflammatory response, e.g.
- Hepatitis*

- Nephritis*
- Suppurative diseases*

Allergies*
Autoimmune polyarthritis
Bullous pemphigoid
Immune-mediated haemolytic anaemia
Immune-mediated thrombocytopenia
Pemphigus complex
Systemic lupus erythematosus
Neoplasia
   Lymphoma

Monoclonal/oligoclonal

Cutaneous amyloidosis
Idiopathic
Macroglobulinaemia
Plasmacytic gastroenterocolitis
Infectious
   Ehrlichiosis
   Leishmaniasis
Neoplastic
   Extramedullary plasmacytoma
   Lymphoma*
   Multiple myeloma

4.1.20   Glucose

Decreased

Polycythaemia *q.v.*
Renal disease* *q.v.*
Sepsis*

Artefact

   Prolonged contact of serum/plasma with erythrocytes

Drugs/toxins

Anabolic steroids
Beta blockers, e.g.
- Propranolol

Ethanol
Ethylene glycol
Insulin
Salicylates
Sulphonylurea
Xylitol

Endocrine
Growth hormone deficiency
Hypoadrenocorticism (D)
Hypopituitarism
Insulinoma

Hepatic
Hepatic failure
- Cirrhosis*
- Hepatic necrosis, e.g.
  - Infection
  - Toxin
  - Trauma
- Portosystemic shunts (acquired or congenital)

Idiopathic
Juvenile
Neonatal

Neoplastic *
Hepatic leiomyoma/leiomyosarcoma
Hepatic/splenic haemangiosarcoma
Hepatocellular carcinoma
Pancreatic

Substrate deficiency
Glycogen storage disease
Hunting dog hypoglycaemia
Juvenile hypoglycaemia
Neonatal hypoglycaemia
Pregnancy hypoglycaemia
Reduced dietary intake of glucose or its precursors, e.g.
- Severe malnutrition
Sepsis

Increased
Excitement
Pancreatitis* (and other pancreatic diseases)
Parenteral nutrition
Postprandial
Renal insufficiency* *q.v.*
Stress hyperglycaemia*
Supplementation, e.g. IV fluids

Artefact
Azotaemia

Drugs/toxins
Daffodil
Ethylene glycol
Glucagon
Glucocorticoids
Hydrochlorothiazide
Ketamine
Megestrol acetate
Oestrogens
Phenytoin
Progestagens
Snake venom
Thiazide diuretics
Xylazine (and other alpha-2 agents)

Endocrine
Acromegaly
Diabetes mellitus*
Hyperadrenocorticism
Hyperpituitarism
Hyperthyroidism
Pheochromocytoma

Progesterone induced*, e.g.
Dioestrus
Lactation
Pregnancy

4.1.21 Iron

Decreased
Acute phase inflammatory reactions*
Chronic inflammatory disease*
Hypothyroidism (D)
Portosystemic shunt
Renal disease* *q.v.*

Chronic external blood loss*, e.g.
Chronically bleeding external masses*
External parasites, e.g.
  • Heavy flea burden*
Gastrointestinal*, e.g.
  • Clotting disorder *q.v.*
  • Neoplasia
  • Parasitism
  • Ulceration

Decreased intake
Milk-only diet in immature animals

Neoplasia
Lymphoma
Osteosarcoma

Increased
Haemolysis* *q.v.*
Ingestion of iron supplements/parenteral overdose
Liver disease* *q.v.*
Refractory anaemia

4.1.22 Lactate dehydrogenase

Increased

Artefact
Haemolysis
Sample ageing

Cardiac muscle disorders
  Degeneration
  Ischaemia
    • Aortic thromboembolism*
    • Bacterial endocarditis
    • Dirofilariasis
    • Myocardial infarction
  Neoplasia
  Trauma

Miscellaneous
  Hepatocellular damage* *q.v.*
  Hyperthyroidism* (C)

*Respiratory disease**
  Necrosis
  Pulmonary thromboembolism

Skeletal muscle disorders
  Exertional rhabdomyolysis
  Neoplasia*
  Seizures*
  Trauma*

Endocrine
  Hyperadrenocorticism*
  Hypothyroidism* (D)

Inflammatory/infectious
  Bacterial*
  Protozoal*

Idiopathic
  Idiopathic polymyositis
  Masticatory myopathy

Inherited myopathies
  Hereditary Labrador retriever myopathy
  Muscular dystrophy
  Myotonia

Metabolic
Glycogen storage diseases
Mitochondrial myopathy

Nutritional
Vitamin E deficiency

Vascular
Aortic thromboembolism* (C)

4.1.23 Lipase

Decreased

Artefact
Haemolysis
Hyperbilirubinaemia
Lipaemia

Increased

Drugs
Azathioprine
Diazoxide
Frusemide
Glucocorticoids
L-Asparaginase
Metronidazole
Oestrogens
Potassium bromide
Sulphonamides
Tetracyclines
Thiazide diuretics

Pancreatic disease
Necrosis
Neoplasia
Pancreatic duct obstruction
Pancreatitis*

Reduced glomerular filtration
  Pre-renal disease* *q.v.*
  Renal disease* *q.v.*
  Post-renal disease* *q.v.*

4.1.24 Triglycerides

Decreased
  Artefact
  • Intravenous dipyrone
  Hyperthyroidism* (C)
  Protein-losing enteropathy*
  Drugs
  • Ascorbic acid therapy

Increased
  Artefact
  • Hyperbilirubinaemia
  Postprandial*

Drugs
  Glucocorticoids
  Megestrol acetate

Primary/idiopathic hyperlipidaemia
  Familial hyperchylomicronaemia in the cat
  Idiopathic hypertriglyceridaemia of the miniature schnauzer
  Idiopathic hypertriglyceridaemia
  Lipoprotein lipase deficiency (C)
  Transient hyperlipidaemia and anaemia in kittens (C)

Secondary hyperlipidaemia
  Acute pancreatitis*
  Cholestasis*
  Diabetes mellitus*
  Hepatic insufficiency* *q.v.*
  Hyperadrenocorticism
  Hypothyroidism* (D)
  Nephrotic syndrome

4.1.25 Troponin

Increased

Cardiac disease, e.g.
Aortic stenosis
Arrhythmogenic right ventricular cardiomyopathy
Bradyarrhythmias
Dilated cardiomyopathy
Mitral valve disease
Pericardial effusion
Pulmonary hypertension
Pulmonic stenosis

Drugs/toxins
Albuterol
Anaesthesia/sedation
Benfluorex
Doxorubicin
Oleander
Phenazopyridine
Phenylpropanolamine
Ractopamine
Viper envenomation

Infections
Babesiosis
Dirofilariasis
Ehrlichiosis
Leishmaniasis
Pyometra

Miscellaneous
Anaemia
Azotaemia/renal disease
Brachycephalic obstructive airway syndrome
Gastric dilatation and volvulus
Heat stroke
Hyperadrenocorticism
Hypoadrenocorticism

   Neoplasia, e.g. lymphoma
   Pancreatitis
   Steroid-responsive meningitis–arteritis

Physiological
   Breed variation (greyhounds)
   High-intensity exercise
   Old age

4.1.26 Trypsin-like immunoreactivity

Decreased
   Exocrine pancreatic insufficiency
   Very-low-protein diet

Increased
   High-protein diet
   Pancreatitis*
   Post-pancreatic obstruction
   Reduced glomerular filtration rate

4.1.27 Urea

Increased

Pre-renal
   Dehydration*
   Gastrointestinal bleeding
   Heart failure*
   High-protein diet*
   Hypoadrenocorticism (D)
   Increased catabolic state, e.g.
     • Fever*
   Shock* *q.v.*
   Tetracyclines

Renal
Acute kidney injury
   Diabetes mellitus*

Drugs/toxins
- ACE inhibitors
- Anaesthetics
- Antibiotics, e.g.
  - Aminoglycosides
  - Amphotericin B
  - Cephalosporins
  - Tetracyclines
- Borax
- Calcium edetate
- Chemotherapeutics, e.g.
  - Cisplatin
- Cimetidine
- Corticosteroids
- Dipyrone (metamizole)
- Heavy metals, e.g.
  - Arsenic
  - Lead
  - Mercury
- Hymenoptera stings
- Intravenous radiographic contrast agents
- Iron/iron salts

Lily ingestion (C)
Melamine toxicity
Methylene blue
- NSAIDs
- Organic compounds, e.g.
  - Ethylene glycol
  - Herbicides
  - Pesticides
- Pigments, e.g.
  - Myoglobin/haemoglobin
  - Paraquat
  - Plastic explosives
  - Salt
  - Snake venom

Hypercalcaemia
Immune-mediated diseases, e.g.
- Glomerulonephritis
- Systemic lupus erythematosus

Infection e.g.
- Leptospirosis
- Pyelonephritis

Ischaemia
- Decreased cardiac output*
- Extensive burns
- Hyper-/hypothermia* *q.v.*
- Prolonged anaesthesia*
- Renal vessel thrombosis
- Shock, e.g.
  - Hypovolaemia
  - Sepsis*
- Transfusion reactions
- Trauma*

Urinary tract obstruction*

Chronic kidney disease, e.g.

Subsequent to acute kidney injury
Glomerulonephritis*
Interstitial nephritis*
Nephrotoxins

Post-renal

Bladder obstruction*, e.g.
- Blood clot
- Neoplasia
- Polyp*
- Urolith*

Bladder trauma
Ureteral obstruction (may need to be bilateral to cause azotaemia)
Urethral obstruction, e.g.
- Neoplasia
- Urolith

Urethral trauma
Uroabdomen

Decreased

Normal in neonates*

Dialysis/over-hydration
Diuresis, e.g.
- Fluid and drug therapy*

Liver insufficiency, e.g.
- Cirrhosis
- Portosystemic shunt*

Low-protein diet/malnutrition*
Polyuria *q.v.*, e.g.
- Diabetes insipidus
- Hyperadrenocorticism

Pregnancy*
Urea cycle enzyme deficiency

4.1.28 Vitamin B12 (cobalamin)

Decreased
Exocrine pancreatic insufficiency
Hepatic lipidosis (C)
Inflammatory biliary tract disorders
Inherited defect of absorption, e.g. border collie
Intestinal mucosal disease*
Pancreatitis

Increased
Vitamin B12 supplementation

4.1.29 Zinc

Decreased
Decreased dietary intake
Zinc-responsive dermatosis

Increased
Ingestion of zinc-containing objects, e.g.
- Coins

4.2 Haematological findings

4.2.1 Regenerative anaemia

HAEMORRHAGE

Internal
Bleeding tumour*
Coagulopathy *q.v.*
Traumatic injury*

External
Bleeding tumour*
Coagulopathy *q.v.*
Epistaxis *q.v.*
Haematemesis *q.v.*
Haematuria *q.v.*
Intestinal blood loss *q.v.*
Traumatic injury*

Parasitism*
Ancylostoma spp.
Fleas
Lice
Ticks
Uncinaria spp.

HAEMOLYSIS

Acquired defects of red cells
Hypophosphataemia

Chemical damage
Copper
Cyclic hydrocarbons
Heavy metals
Propylene glycol

Oxidative damage (Heinz body anaemia)
Benzocaine toxicity
DL-methionine toxicity

Garlic toxicity
Glycol toxicity
High doses of vitamin K
Lymphoma
Metabolic disease
- Diabetes mellitus*
- Hyperthyroidism* (C)
- Renal disease*
Methylene blue
Onion toxicity
Paracetamol toxicity
Phenazopyridine (C)
Phenolic compound toxicity, e.g.
- Mothballs
Propylene toxicity
Vitamin K3 toxicity
Zinc toxicity

Genetic defects of red cells
Feline porphyria
Hereditary elliptocytosis
Hereditary haemolysis in Abyssinian and Somali cats (C)
Hereditary stomatocytosis
Methaemoglobin reductase deficiency
Non-spherocytic haemolytic anaemia of beagles (D)
Phosphofructokinase deficiency (D)
Pyruvate kinase deficiency

Immune mediated
Primary (autoimmune haemolytic anaemia)*

Drugs/toxins
Anti-arrhythmics
Anticonvulsants
Bee envenomation
Cephalosporins
Chlorpromazine
Copper
Dipyrone
Levamisole
Methimazole

Methylene blue
NSAIDs, e.g.
  • Paracetamol
Penicillins
Propylthiouracil
Quinidine
Trimethoprim/sulphonamide

Immunological
Anti-lymphocyte globulin therapy
Neonatal isoerythrolysis
Systemic lupus erythematosus
Transfusion reactions

Infectious
Ancylostoma spp.
Babesiosis
Cytauxzoonosis
Dirofilariasis
Ehrlichiosis
Feline leukaemia virus* (C)
Haemobartonellosis
Leishmaniasis
Leptospirosis*
Trypanosomiasis (D)
Uncinaria spp.

Neoplastic
Haemangiosarcoma
Lymphoproliferative disease, e.g.
  • Leukaemia
  • Lymphoma*

Mechanical injury of red cells
Dirofilariasis
Disseminated intravascular coagulation*
Enlarged spleen
Glomerulonephritis
Haemolytic–uraemic syndrome

Neoplasia causing microangiopathic haemolytic anaemia, e.g.
- Splenic haemangiosarcoma*

Patent ductus arteriosus

Vasculitis

4.2.2 Poorly/non-regenerative anaemia

Normal
Young animals

Acute, pre-regenerative anaemia

Anaemia of chronic disease/associated with systemic disease
Chronic inflammatory disease*
Chronic kidney disease* *q.v.*
Cytauxzoonosis
Feline immunodeficiency virus* (C)
Feline infectious peritonitis* (C)
Feline leukaemia virus* (C)
Hepatic disease* *q.v.*
Histoplasmosis
Hypoadrenocorticism (D)
Hypothyroidism* (D)
Leishmaniasis
Malignant neoplasia
Trypanosomiasis (D)

Bone marrow disorders – reduced red cell production

Aplastic anaemia
Drugs/toxins
- Albendazole
- Anti-cancer chemotherapeutics
- Chloramphenicol
- Cyclic hydrocarbons
- DDT
- Diazoxide
- Oestrogens
- Phenylbutazone
- Sulpha drugs

- Trichloroethylene
- Trimethoprim/sulphadiazine

Hyperoestrogenism, e.g.
- Iatrogenic
- Sertoli cell tumour

Infection
- Ehrlichiosis
- Viruses, e.g.
  - Feline leukaemia virus* (C)
  - Parvovirus*

Irradiation

Haematopoietic neoplasia

Lymphoproliferative
- Lymphoid leukaemia
  - Acute lymphoblastic leukaemia
  - Chronic lymphocytic leukaemia
- Granular lymphocytic leukaemia
- Lymphoma
- Multiple myeloma

Myeloproliferative
- Acute monocytic leukaemia
- Acute myeloid leukaemia
- Acute myelomonocytic leukaemia
- Chronic myeloid/granulocytic leukaemia

Myelodysplasia

Primary
Secondary
- Cobalamin or folate deficiencies
- Drug-induced toxicosis
- Immune-mediated diseases
- Neoplastic diseases

Myelophthisis

Granulomatous inflammation
- Fungi
- Histoplasmosis
- Tuberculosis

Myelofibrosis
- Idiopathic
- Lymphoproliferative
- Myeloproliferative
- Other types of neoplasia
- Prolonged marrow stimulation, e.g.
  - Chronic haemolytic anaemia
- Radiation

Neoplasia
- Leukaemia
- Metastatic neoplasia, e.g.
  - Carcinoma
  - Melanoma

Pure red cell aplasia
Feline leukaemia virus* (C)
Immune mediated

Defects in haemoglobin synthesis

Copper deficiency
Erythropoietic porphyria
Hereditary porphyria
Iron deficiency anaemia *q.v.*
Lead poisoning
Vitamin B6 deficiency

Defects in nucleotide synthesis

Nutrient deficiencies
Cobalt
Folic acid
Vitamin B12

Erythropoietin deficiency

Chronic kidney disease* *q.v.*

Iron deficiency

Inadequate intake
Dietary deficiency, e.g.
- Milk diet

Inadequate stores
  Neonates*

Chronic external haemorrhage
  Bleeding tumour*
  Coagulopathy *q.v.*
  Epistaxis *q.v.*
  Haematemesis *q.v.*
  Haematuria *q.v.*
  Intestinal blood loss *q.v.*
  Parasitism*
  - *Ancylostoma* spp.
  - Fleas
  - Lice
  - Ticks
  - *Uncinaria* spp.

Rapid erythropoiesis
  Erythropoietin therapy of anaemia
  Neonates

Repeat phlebotomy
  Blood donors*
  Frequent blood sampling of small patients*
  Therapeutic phlebotomy, e.g.
  - Polycythaemia

Traumatic injury
  Sideroblastic anaemia

4.2.3 Polycythaemia

Relative polycythaemia

*Dehydration**
  Burns
  Diarrhoea
  Heat stroke
  Polyuria without matching polydipsia

Vomiting
Water deprivation

Splenic contraction *
Excitement
Exercise
Stress

Primary polycythaemia
Myeloproliferative disease (polycythaemia vera/primary erythrocytosis)

Secondary polycythaemia
Physiologically appropriate
Altitude
Chronic respiratory disease, e.g.
- Feline asthma*
- Interstitial fibrosis
- Neoplasia*

Haemoglobinopathies
Right-to-left congenital cardiac shunt, e.g.
- Atrial septal defect with pulmonic stenosis
- Pulmonary arteriovenous fistula
- Reverse-shunting patent ductus arteriosus
- Reverse-shunting ventricular septal defect
- Tetralogy of Fallot

Physiologically inappropriate
Extra-renal neoplasia
- Caecal leiomyosarcoma
- Hepatic carcinoma
- Hepatoblastoma
- Nasal fibrosarcoma

Hyperadrenocorticism
Hyperthyroidism* (C)
Non-neoplastic renal diseases
- Fatty infiltration of the kidney
- Hydronephrosis
- Renal capsular effusion
- Renal cysts

Renal neoplasia
- Adenocarcinoma
- Fibrosarcoma
- Lymphoma
- Nephroblastoma

Toxins, e.g.
- Carbamate

4.2.4 Thrombocytopenia

Decreased production

Bone marrow neoplasia, e.g.
Lymphoproliferative disease
Metastatic disease
Myeloproliferative disease

Drugs
Albendazole
Antibiotics, e.g.
- Chloramphenicol
- Trimethoprim/sulphonamide

Chemotherapeutic/cytotoxic drugs
Chloramphenicol
Diazoxide
Griseofulvin
Methimazole
Oestrogens
Phenylbutazone
Phenytoin
Propylthiouracil
Ribavirin
Thiazide diuretics

Infection
Bacterial
- Endotoxaemia*

Fungal
- Blastomycosis
- Coccidioidomycosis

- Cryptococcosis
- Histoplasmosis

Parasitic

- Cytauxzoonosis
- Hepatozoonosis

Rickettsial

- Ehrlichiosis
- Rocky Mountain spotted fever

Viral

- Canine distemper virus* (D)
- Canine parvovirus* (D)
- Feline immunodeficiency virus* (C)
- Feline infectious enteritis* (C)
- Feline leukaemia virus* (C)

Miscellaneous

Haemophagocytic syndrome
Myelofibrosis

- Idiopathic
- Neoplasia, e.g.
  - Myeloproliferative disease
- Prolonged marrow stimulation
- Secondary to sepsis

Immune-mediated destruction

Primary immune-mediated thrombocytopenia
Concurrent immune-mediated thrombocytopenia and
    immune-mediated haemolytic anaemia (Evans syndrome)

Drugs/toxins

Cephalosporins
Chlorpromazine
Colchicine
Cytotoxic drugs
Dipyrone
Heparin
Levamisole
Methimazole
Modified live vaccines
NSAIDs

Oestrogens
Penicillins
Propylthiouracil
Quinidine
Trimethoprim/sulphonamide

Secondary immune-mediated thrombocytopenia
  Infections
    • Babesiosis
    • Dirofilariasis
    • Ehrlichiosis
    • Feline immunodeficiency virus* (C)
    • Feline leukaemia virus* (C)
    • Leptospirosis
  Neonatal alloimmune thrombocytopenia
  Neoplasia, e.g.
    • Lymphoma*
    • Solid tumours
  Systemic lupus erythematosus
  Transfusion reactions

Increased utilisation/non-immune destruction
Disseminated intravascular coagulation
Haemolytic–uraemic syndrome
Microangiopathic destruction
Septicaemia
Snake venom

Chronic/severe haemorrhage
  Coagulopathy
  Neoplasia

Vasculitis
  Canine adenovirus-1
  Canine herpesvirus
  Dirofilariasis
  Ehrlichiosis
  Feline infectious peritonitis* (C)
  Neoplasia
  Polyarteritis nodosa

Rocky Mountain spotted fever
Septicaemia
Systemic lupus erythematosus

Sequestration
Hepatomegaly* *q.v.*
Sepsis*
Splenomegaly* *q.v.*
- Chronic infection*
- Haematoma*
- Immune-mediated haemolytic anaemia*
- Neoplasia
  - Haemangioma
  - Haemangiosarcoma
  - Mast cell
  - Metastatic
- Portal hypertension
- Splenic torsion
- Splenitis
- Systemic lupus erythematosus

4.2.5 Thrombocytosis

Normal
May be normal in older animals

Splenic contraction
Excitement*
Exercise*
Stress*

Post splenectomy
Primary
Essential thrombocytosis

Reactive
Bradycardia *q.v.*
Chronic haemorrhage* *q.v.*

Fractures*
Gastrointestinal disease* *q.v.*
Hyperadrenocorticism
Hypercoagulability/disseminated intravascular coagulation
Hyperviscosity syndromes
Hypotension*
Infection
Inflammation/immune-mediated disease*
Metastatic carcinoma
Non-specific bone marrow stimulation
Paraneoplastic
- Bronchoalveolar carcinoma
- Chronic myeloid leukaemia
- Gingival carcinoma
- Metastatic squamous cell carcinoma
- Osteosarcoma

Polycythaemia *q.v.*
Shock* *q.v.*

Rebound
Secondary to resolution of previous thrombocytopenia

4.2.6   Neutrophilia

Immunodeficiency syndromes, e.g.
Canine leukocyte adhesion deficiency (D)
Weimaraner immunodeficiency (D)

Inflammatory conditions – acute or chronic*, e.g.
Chemical exposure

Immune-mediated disease, e.g.
Haemolytic anaemia*
Polyarthritis
Systemic lupus erythematosus

Infections
Bacterial*
Fungal
Protozoal
Viral*

Neoplasia
    Necrosis*
    Secondary bacterial infection*
    Ulceration*

Tissue necrosis, e.g.
    Large tumours*
    Pancreatitis*
    Pansteatitis

Toxins
    Endotoxin*
    Snakebite

Physiological
    Stress
    • Adrenaline release
    • Corticosteroid (endogenous or exogenous)

Primary
    Myeloproliferative disease
    • Acute myeloid leukaemia
    • Chronic myeloid leukaemia

Reactive
    Haemolysis* *q.v.*
    Haemorrhage*
    Neoplasia*
    Oestrogen toxicity
    Recent surgery*
    Trauma*

4.2.7 Neutropenia

Decreased neutrophil survival
    Haemophagocytic syndromes
    Immune-mediated neutropenia (D)
    Parvovirus enteritis*

Sepsis/endotoxaemia*, e.g.
  Acute salmonellosis*
  Aspiration pneumonia*
  Peritonitis*
  Pyometra*
  Pyothorax*

Reduced neutrophil release
Trapped neutrophil syndrome in border collie (D)

Reduced neutrophil production
  Canine cyclic haematopoiesis

Acute viral infections*
  Canine parvovirus* (D)
  Feline immunodeficiency virus* (C)
  Feline leukaemia virus* (C)
  Feline panleukopenia virus* (C)
  Infectious canine hepatitis* (D)

Bone marrow disease
  Aplastic anaemia
    • Ehrlichiosis
    • Idiopathic
    • Toxicity
      ◦ Oestrogen
      ◦ Phenylbutazone
  Bone marrow neoplasia, e.g.
    • Lymphoproliferative disease
    • Metastatic neoplasia
    • Myeloproliferative disease
  Disseminated granulomatous disease
  Immune-mediated destruction of neutrophil precursors
  Myelodysplasia
  Myelophthisis

Bone marrow suppression
  Drugs
    • Albendazole
    • Azathioprine
    • Busulphan

- Carbimazole
- Carboplatin
- Chlorambucil
- Chloramphenicol
- Cyclophosphamide
- Cytarabine
- Diazoxide
- Doxorubicin
- Frusemide
- Griseofulvin
- Hydroxyurea
- Lomustine
- Melphalan
- Methimazole
- Oestrogen
- Phenobarbitone
- Phenylbutazone
- Trimethoprim/sulphonamide (C)
- Vinblastine

Oestrogen toxicity, e.g.
- Iatrogenic
- Sertoli cell tumour

Radiation therapy

4.2.8 Lymphocytosis

Miscellaneous
Chronic infection*
Hypoadrenocorticism (D)
Recent vaccination*

Neoplasia
Leukaemia
- Acute lymphoblastic leukaemia
- Chronic lymphocytic leukaemia

Stage V lymphoma

Physiological*
Excitement*
Exercise*

Immature animal*
Post vaccination*
Stress (adrenaline response)*

4.2.9   Lymphopenia

Drugs
Albendazole
Azathioprine
Busulphan
Carbimazole
Carboplatin
Chlorambucil
Chloramphenicol
Corticosteroids
Cyclophosphamide
Cyclosporin
Cytarabine
Diazoxide
Doxorubicin
Frusemide
Griseofulvin
Hydroxyurea
Lomustine
Melphalan
Phenylbutazone
Trimethoprim/sulphonamide (C)
Vinblastine

Endocrine
Hyperadrenocorticism

Immunodeficiency syndromes, e.g.
Basset hound
Cardigan Welsh corgi
Jack Russell terrier

Infectious/inflammatory
Septicaemia*

Viral infections, e.g.
Canine distemper virus* (D)
Coronavirus*
Feline immunodeficiency virus* (C)
Feline leukaemia virus* (C)
Infectious canine hepatitis* (D)
Parvovirus

Loss of lymph
Chylothorax
Lymphangiectasia
Protein-losing enteropathy* *q.v.*

Physiological
Stress (corticosteroid response)*

4.2.10   Monocytosis

Chronic inflammation
Granulomatous inflammation
Pyogranulomatous inflammation
Suppuration*
Tissue necrosis*

Corticosteroids
Hyperadrenocorticism
Iatrogenic
Stress

Infections

Fungal, e.g.
Coccidioidomycosis

Parasitic, e.g.
Leishmaniasis

Viral, e.g.
Feline immunodeficiency virus* (C)

Bacterial e.g.
  Rickettsial

Haemolytic/haemorrhagic diseases* q.v.

Immune-mediated disease, e.g.
  Immune-mediated haemolytic anaemia*
  Immune-mediated polyarthritis

Neoplasia
  Monocytic leukaemia
  Myelomonocytic leukaemia
  Tumours with necrotic centres*

4.2.11   Eosinophilia

Hormonal
  Hypoadrenocorticism
  Oestrus in some bitches

Immune mediated
  Allergies *
    • Atopy*
    • Feline asthma* (C)
    • Flea allergy*
    • Food allergies*
  Canine panosteitis (D)
  Eosinophilic bronchopneumopathy (D)
  Eosinophilic gastroenteritis*
  Eosinophilic granuloma complex*
  Eosinophilic myositis
  Feline hypereosinophilic syndrome (C)
  Pemphigus foliaceus

Infection

*Bacterial**

Fungal, e.g.
  Aspergillosis
  Cryptococcosis

Parasites*, e.g.
  Aelurostrongylus abstrusus
  Ancylostoma spp.
  Angiostrongylus vasorum
  Capillaria aerophila
  Dirofilaria immitis
  Oslerus osleri
  Pneumonyssoides caninum
  Trichuris vulpis

Neoplastic
  Eosinophilic leukaemia

Tumour-associated eosinophilia
  Fibrosarcoma
  Myeloproliferative disease
  Lymphoma
  Mast cell tumour
  Mucinous carcinomas
  Transitional cell carcinoma

4.2.12 Eosinopenia

  Acute infection*
  Acute inflammation*
  Bone marrow aplasia/hypoplasia
  Glucocorticoid therapy*
  Hyperadrenocorticism
  Stress*

4.2.13 Mastocytemia

  Disseminated mast cell neoplasia
  Mast cell leukaemia
  Mast cell tumour*, e.g.
  • Intestinal tract
  • Spleen
  Severe inflammation

4.2.14   Basophilia

Chronic granulocytic leukaemia
Hyperlipoproteinaemia
Hypersensitivity reactions
Lymphoma
Lymphomatoid granulomatosis
Lymphoplasmacytic gastroenteritis
Mast cell tumours*
Parasitism, especially dirofilariasis

4.2.15   Increased buccal mucosal bleeding time (disorders of primary haemostasis)

Thrombocytopenia q.v.

Thrombocytopathia

Acquired

Chronic anaemia
Disseminated intravascular coagulation
Drugs/toxins
- Antibiotics
- Barbiturates
- Calcium channel blockers
- Colloids
- Heparin
- Hetastarch
- NSAIDs, especially aspirin
- Propranolol
- Theophylline
- Snake venom

Hepatic disease*
Infection
- Ehrlichiosis
- Feline leukaemia virus* (C)

Neoplasia*, e.g.
- Lymphocytic leukaemia
- Multiple myeloma

Paraproteinaemias
- Benign macroglobulinaemia
- Polyclonal gammopathies

Uraemia* *q.v.*

Inherited

Basset hound thrombopathia (D)
Canine thrombasthenic thrombopathia of otter hounds
and great pyrenees (D)
Chédiak–Higashi syndrome (C)
Cocker spaniel bleeding disorders (D)
Cyclic haematopoiesis (grey collie)
Glanzmann's thrombasthenia (D)
von Willebrand's disease* (D)

4.2.16   Increased prothrombin time (disorders of extrinsic and common pathways)

Artefact
Deficiency of factor II, V, VII or X
Disseminated intravascular coagulation
Hypo- or dysfibrinogenaemia
Liver disease*, e.g.
- Portosystemic shunt
- Vitamin K antagonism*

4.2.17   Increased partial thromboplastin time or activated clotting time (disorders of intrinsic and common pathways)

Colloid administration
Disseminated intravascular coagulation
Factor II, V, X, XI or XII deficiency
Haemophilia A (factor VIII deficiency)
Haemophilia B (factor IX deficiency)
Haemorrhage
Hypo- or dysfibrinogenaemia

Liver disease* *q.v.*
Vitamin K antagonism*
Vitamin K-dependent coagulopathy

4.2.18   Increased fibrin degradation products

Disseminated intravascular coagulation
Hepatic disease* *q.v.*
Hyperfibrinogenolysis
Internal haemorrhage
Thrombosis*
Vitamin K antagonism*

4.2.19   Decreased fibrinogen levels

Artefact
- Clot
- Incorrect anticoagulant

Disseminated intravascular coagulation*
Excessive blood loss*
Hereditary fibrinogen deficiency
Immune-mediated haemolytic anaemia
Severe hepatic deficiency

4.2.20   Decreased antithrombin III levels

Heparin therapy
Hepatic disease* *q.v.*
Hypercoagulability, e.g.
- Disseminated intravascular coagulation

Protein-losing enteropathy* *q.v.*, e.g.
- Parvovirus enteritis

Protein-losing nephropathy* *q.v.*

4.3   Electrolyte and blood gas findings

4.3.1   Total calcium

Decreased
Acute pancreatitis*
Acute kidney injury *q.v.*
Canine distemper virus* (D)
Chronic kidney disease* *q.v.*
Exocrine pancreatic insufficiency (D)
Hypoalbuminaemia* *q.v.*
Hypomagnesaemia *q.v.*
Hypoproteinaemia
Hypovitaminosis D
Iatrogenic (post thyroidectomy)*
Idiopathic
Infarction of parathyroid gland adenomas
Intestinal malabsorption*
Lactational hypocalcaemia
Medullary carcinoma of the thyroid (C-cell tumour)
Nutritional secondary hyperparathyroidism
Primary hypoparathyroidism
Puerperal tetany (eclampsia)*
Rhabdomyolysis
Tumour lysis syndrome

Artefact
Haemolysis
Incorrect anticoagulant

Drugs/toxins
Anticonvulsants
Calcitonin therapy
EDTA
Ethylene glycol
Frusemide
Glucagon
Intravenous phosphate administration

Mithramycin
Oxalate toxicity
Pamidronate
Phosphate-containing enemas
Sodium bicarbonate
Transfusion using citrated blood

Increased

Acute kidney injury *q.v.*
Artefact
- Lipaemia

Chronic kidney disease* *q.v.*
Dehydration/hyperalbuminaemia* *q.v.*
Granulomatous disease
Hypervitaminosis A
Hypervitaminosis D
Hypoadrenocorticism (D)
Idiopathic hypercalcaemia of cats (C)
Physiological
- Postprandial
- Young dog*

Tertiary hyperparathyroidism

Drugs/toxins

Anabolic steroids
Calcipotriol
Cholecalciferol rodenticides
Hydralazine
Jasmine
Oestrogen
Oral or intravenous calcium
Oral phosphate binders
Paracetamol
Parenteral calcium administration
Progesterone
Testosterone
Trilostane
Vitamin D analogues

Hypercalcaemia of malignancy

Carcinoma
- Bronchogenic
- Mammary
- Nasal cavity
- Prostatic
- Squamous cell
- Thyroid

Haematological malignancies
- Lymphoma*
- Multiple myeloma
- Myeloproliferative disease

Metastatic or primary bone neoplasia *q.v.*

Pseudohyperparathyroidism
- Apocrine gland adenocarcinoma*
- Lymphoma*

Primary hyperparathyroidism

Hereditary neonatal hyperparathyroidism
Multiple endocrine neoplasia
Parathyroid gland adenoma
Parathyroid gland carcinoma
Primary hyperplasia of the parathyroid glands

Skeletal lesions

Bone metastases
Hypertrophic osteodystrophy
Osteomyelitis
Systemic mycoses

4.3.2 Chloride

Note: Most causes of hyperchloraemia also cause concurrent hypernatraemia, and if changes are proportionate, it is usually easier to look for causes of hypernatraemia. Formulae to correct chloride to account for sodium changes have been suggested as follows:

Dogs: Cl^- (corrected) = Cl^- (measured) $\times [146 / Na^+$ (measured)]

     Reference ranges: Cl^- (measured) = $100 - 116$ mmol / l

                            Cl^- (corrected) = $107 - 113$ mmol / l

Cats: Cl^- (corrected) = Cl^- (measured) $\times [156 / Na^+$ (measured)]

     Reference ranges: Cl^- (measured) = $100 - 124$ mmol / l

                            Cl^- (corrected) = $117 - 123$ mmol / l

Note: Reference ranges may vary depending on the instruments used to perform the measurement.

Decreased

Artefact
    Lipaemia

Corrected hypochloraemia
    Chronic respiratory acidosis *q.v.*
    Exercise*
    Hyperadrenocorticism
    Vomiting*
    Drugs
       • Frusemide
       • Sodium bicarbonate
       • Thiazide diuretics

Increased

Artefact
    Hypotonic water loss
    Lipaemia
    Potassium bromide therapy
    Pure water loss

Corrected hyperchloraemia
    Chronic respiratory alkalosis *q.v.*
    Diabetes mellitus*
    Drugs/toxins
       • Acetazolamide
       • Fluid therapy with saline

- Potassium chloride supplementation
- Salt poisoning
- Spironolactone
- Total parenteral nutrition
- Urinary acidifiers, e.g. ammonium chloride

Fanconi syndrome
Hyperaldosteronism
Hypoadrenocorticism (D)
Renal disease* *q.v.*
Renal tubular acidosis
Small intestinal diarrhoea*

4.3.3 Magnesium

Decreased
Acute pancreatitis*
Cholestasis* *q.v.*
Decreased intake
Hypercalcaemia *q.v.*
Hypokalaemia *q.v.*

Artefact
Haemolysis

Drugs/iatrogenic
Amino acids
Aminoglycosides
Blood transfusion
Cisplatin
Digitalis
Diuretics, e.g.
- Frusemide
- Thiazides

Haemodialysis
Insulin
Nasogastric suction
Pamidronate
Peritoneal dialysis

Prolonged intravenous fluid therapy
Total parenteral nutrition

Endocrine
Diabetic ketoacidosis*
Hyperthyroidism* (C)
Hypoparathyroidism (ionised
hypomagnesaemia)
Primary hyperaldosteronism
Primary hyperparathyroidism

Intestinal loss
Bowel resection
Enteropathies*

Redistribution
Hypothermia* *q.v.*
Sepsis*
Trauma*

Renal
Acute tubular necrosis
Drug-induced tubular injury
  • Aminoglycosides
  • Cisplatin
Post-obstructive diuresis*

Increased
Artefact
  • Sample haemolysis
Drugs
  • Oral antacids
  • Parenteral administration
  • Progesterones
Haemolysis
Hypoadrenocorticism (D)
Obstructive uropathy*
Renal disease* *q.v.*
Thoracic neoplasia/pleural effusion (C)

4.3.4 Potassium

Decreased

Diet
Decreased dietary intake
High-protein acidifying diets

Drugs/iatrogenic
Albuterol
Amphotericin B
Catecholamines
Dialysis
Diuretics, e.g.
- Frusemide
- Mineralocorticoids
- Penicillins
- Thiazides
Fludrocortisone
Frusemide
Glucose
Hydrochlorothiazide
Inadequate potassium supplementation during fluid therapy
Insulin
Terbutaline
Total parenteral nutrition

Endocrine
Diabetes mellitus*
Hyperadrenocorticism
Mineralocorticoid excess
Primary hyperaldosteronism

Increased loss
Chronic kidney disease* *q.v.*
Diuresis, e.g.
- Diabetes mellitus*
- Diuretic therapy
Gastrointestinal loss (vomiting, diarrhoea)* *q.v.*

Post-obstructive diuresis*
Renal tubular acidosis

Translocation
Alkalosis
Hypothermia* *q.v.*
Idiopathic hypokalaemia of Burmese cats (C)

Increased

Artefact/pseudohyperkalaemia
Contamination of sample with potassium EDTA
Haemolysis (especially Japanese Akita)
Marked leukocytosis/thrombocytosis with delay
in separating serum
Thrombocytosis

Decreased urinary excretion
Acute kidney injury *q.v.*
Repeated drainage of effusions, e.g. chylothorax
Gastrointestinal diseases*
- Perforated duodenal ulcer
- Salmonellosis
- Trichuriasis
Hyporeninaemic hypoaldosteronism
Post-renal failure* *q.v.*
Ruptured bladder/uroperitoneum
Hypoadrenocorticism (D)

Drugs/toxins
ACE inhibitors
Amiloride
Beta blockers
Cardiac glycosides
Ethylene glycol
NSAIDs
Oral or parenteral potassium supplementation
Paraquat
Prostaglandin inhibitors
Salbutamol
Spironolactone

Succinylcholine
Tricyclic antidepressants
Trilostane

Increased intake
Iatrogenic

Translocation
Acidosis *q.v.*
Diabetes mellitus/diabetic ketoacidosis*
Reperfusion injury, e.g.
  • Aortic thromboembolism
  • Crush
Tumour lysis syndrome

4.3.5 Phosphate

Decreased

Decreased dietary intake
Decreased intestinal absorption
Diarrhoea* *q.v.*
Eclampsia*
Hypercalcaemia of malignancy*
Hypothermia* *q.v.*
Hypovitaminosis D
Increased urinary excretion*
Metabolic acidosis* *q.v.*
Renal tubular defects, e.g.
  • Fanconi syndrome
Respiratory alkalosis *q.v.*
Vomiting* *q.v.*

Drugs/iatrogenic
Bicarbonate
Diuretics
Fluid therapy
Glucocorticoids
Glucose
Insulin

Pamidronate
Phosphate-binding antacids
Salicylates
Vitamin D deficiency

Endocrine disorders
Diabetic ketoacidosis*
Hyperadrenocorticism
Hyperinsulinism/insulinoma
Primary hyperparathyroidism

Increased

Acute kidney injury or chronic kidney
disease* *q.v.*
Haemolysis* *q.v.*
Metabolic acidosis* *q.v.*
Muscle trauma/necrosis*
Normal juvenile animal
Osteolytic bone lesions
Pre-renal azotaemia* *q.v.*
Post-renal azotaemia *q.v.*
Tumour lysis syndrome

Artefact
Haemolysis

Drugs/toxins
Cholecalciferol rodenticides
Hypervitaminosis D
Jasmine toxicity
Phosphate-containing enemas
Phosphate supplementation

Endocrine disorders
Acromegaly
Hyperthyroidism* (C)
Nutritional secondary hyperparathyroidism
Primary hypoparathyroidism
Renal secondary hyperparathyroidism*

4.3.6 Sodium

Decreased

Congestive heart failure with effusion*
Diarrhoea*
Hyperglycaemia* *q.v.*
Hyperlipidaemia *q.v.*
Hypoadrenocorticism (D)
Inappropriate antidiuretic hormone secretion
Inappropriate fluid therapy
Liver disease with ascites* *q.v.*
Marked hyperproteinaemia *q.v.*
Myxoedema coma of hypothyroidism
Nephrotic syndrome with effusion
Over-hydration
Pancreatitis*
Psychogenic polydipsia*
Renal disease* *q.v.*
Vomiting* *q.v.*

Dehydration/hypovolaemia

Cutaneous loss, e.g.
  • Burns
Gastrointestinal loss*
Hypoadrenocorticism (D)

Drugs

Cyclophosphamide
Diuretics, e.g.
  • Amiloride
  • Frusemide
  • Mannitol
  • Spironolactone
  • Thiazides
NSAIDs
Vincristine

Effusions

Peritonitis*

Pleural effusion* *q.v.*
Uroabdomen

Third space loss
Chylothorax with repeated drainage
Pancreatitis*
Peritonitis*
Uroabdomen

Increased

Drugs/toxins
Fludrocortisone
Hypertonic saline
Salt-containing products, e.g.
* Playdough
Sodium bicarbonate
Sodium phosphate enemas

Hypotonic fluid loss
Cutaneous, e.g.
* Burns
Diabetes mellitus (secondary to osmotic diuresis)*
Gastrointestinal (vomiting, diarrhoea, small intestinal obstruction)* *q.v.*
Post-obstructive diuresis*
Renal disease* *q.v.*
Third space loss, e.g.
* Pancreatitis*
* Peritonitis*

Increased intake
Hyperadrenocorticism
Hyperaldosteronism
Iatrogenic
Salt poisoning

Pure water loss
Hypodipsia or adipsia, e.g.
* Cranial trauma
* Diabetes insipidus

- Inflammatory brain disease
- Intracranial neoplasia

Hyperthermia *q.v.*

Lack of free access to water with normal or increased insensible losses

Panting/hyperventilation

Severe exercise in greyhounds

4.3.7 pH

ACIDAEMIA

Metabolic acidosis

Diabetic ketoacidosis*

Hypoadrenocorticism (D)

Post-hypocapnic metabolic acidosis

Renal disease* *q.v.*

Renal tubular acidosis

Drugs/toxins

Acetazolamide

Ammonium chloride

Ethylene glycol

Methanol

Methionine

Paraldehyde

Salicylic acid

Lactic acid production

Diarrhoea* *q.v.*

Hypoxaemia

Pancreatitis*

Sepsis*

Shock* *q.v.*

Respiratory acidosis

Cardiopulmonary arrest

CNS disease (brainstem/high cervical spinal lesion), e.g.

Intracranial space-occupying lesion

Trauma

Iatrogenic respiratory depression
  Anaesthesia
  Opiates
  Organophosphates
  Pancuronium
  Succinylcholine

Neuromuscular defects
  Botulism
  Idiopathic hypokalaemia of Burmese cats (C)
  Myasthenia gravis
  Polymyositis
  Polyradiculoneuritis
  Tetanus
  Tick paralysis

Severe respiratory disease
  Acute respiratory distress syndrome
  Airway obstruction*
  Aspiration pneumonia
  Chest wall trauma
  Diaphragmatic hernia*
  Haemothorax*
  Neoplasia*
  Pleural effusion* *q.v.*
  Pneumonia* *q.v.*
  Pneumothorax* *q.v.*
  Pulmonary fibrosis
  Pulmonary oedema* *q.v.*
  Pulmonary thromboembolism
  Pyothorax*
  Smoke inhalation

ALKALAEMIA

Metabolic alkalosis
  Hyperadrenocorticism
  Post hypercapnia
  Primary hyperaldosteronism
  Vomiting*

Drugs
  Acetate
  Bicarbonate
  Citrate
  Diuretics
  Exogenous steroid therapy
  Gluconate
  Lactate

Respiratory alkalosis
  Overzealous ventilator therapy

Direct stimulation of medullary respiratory centre (neurogenic hyperventilation)
  CNS disease *q.v.*
  Hepatic disease *q.v.*
  Sepsis*
  Drugs
  • Methyl xanthines
  • Salicylate intoxication

Hypoxaemia, e.g.
  Congestive heart failure*
  High altitude
  Pulmonary disease*
  Right-to-left cardiac shunts
  Severe anaemia* *q.v.*

Panting/hyperventilation
  Anxiety*
  Fever*
  Heat stroke*
  Hyperthyroidism* (C)
  Pain*

4.3.8 paO2

Decreased

CNS disease (brainstem/high cervical spinal lesion), e.g.
  Intracranial space-occupying lesion
  Trauma

Heart disease
Pulmonary oedema* *q.v.*
Right-to-left shunting

Iatrogenic respiratory depression
Anaesthesia
Opiates
Organophosphates
Pancuronium
Succinylcholine

Inadequate oxygen in inspired air
Failure of oxygen supply during anaesthesia
High altitude

Neuromuscular defects
Botulism
Idiopathic hypokalaemia of Burmese cats (C)
Myasthenia gravis
Polymyositis
Polyradiculoneuritis
Tetanus
Tick paralysis

Severe respiratory disease
Acute respiratory distress syndrome
Airway obstruction*
Aspiration pneumonia*
Chest wall trauma*
Diaphragmatic hernia*
Haemothorax*
Neoplasia*
Pleural effusion* *q.v.*
Pneumonia* *q.v.*
Pneumothorax* *q.v.*
Pulmonary fibrosis
Pulmonary oedema* *q.v.*
Pulmonary thromboembolism
Pyothorax*
Smoke inhalation

Increased
Oxygen supplementation

4.3.9   Total CO2

Decreased
Respiratory alkalosis *q.v.*

Increased
Respiratory acidosis *q.v.*

4.3.10   Bicarbonate

Decreased
Metabolic acidosis *q.v.*

Increased
Metabolic alkalosis *q.v.*

4.3.11   Base excess

Decreased
Metabolic acidosis *q.v.*

Increased
Metabolic alkalosis *q.v.*

4.4   Urinalysis findings

4.4.1   Alterations in specific gravity

HYPOSTHENURIA
Increased water loss but no increased loss of solutes

Drugs
Anticonvulsants
Carbonic anhydrase inhibitors

Corticosteroids
Frusemide
Spironolactone
Thiazide diuretics

Polyuria due to decreased ADH secretion
Drugs, e.g.
- Adrenaline
- Phenytoin
Insulinoma
Over-hydration
Pheochromocytoma
Primary central diabetes insipidus
Psychogenic polydipsia*

Polyuria due to ADH inhibition/resistance
Hyperadrenocorticism
Hypercalcaemia* *q.v.*
Hyperthyroidism* (C)
Hypokalaemia* *q.v.*
Liver disease* *q.v.*
Primary hyperparathyroidism
Primary nephrogenic diabetes insipidus
Toxaemia, e.g.
- Pyometra*

Inability of kidneys to concentrate urine
Acute kidney injury *q.v.*
Chronic kidney disease* *q.v.*
Hypoadrenocorticism (loss of medullary concentrating gradient)
Pyelonephritis

HYPERSTHENURIA
Polyuria with excess solute loss
Acromegaly
Diabetes mellitus*
Diet
- High protein
- High salt

Fanconi syndrome
Hyperviscosity
Osmotic diuretics
- Dextrose
- Mannitol
Primary renal glucosuria

Decreased loss of water and no decreased loss of solutes

Cardiac failure*
Dehydration*
Haemorrhage*
Renal infarction
Shock* *q.v.*

4.4.2   Abnormalities in urine chemistry

Bilirubin

False positive, e.g. pigmenturia
Fever* *q.v.*
Haemolytic disease
Hyperbilirubinaemia* *q.v.*
Normal in small quantities in dogs*
Starvation*

Blood

See Haematuria *q.v.*

Glucose

Hyperglycaemia q.v.
Diabetes mellitus*
Hyperadrenocorticism
Iatrogenic
Pheochromocytoma
Primary hyperaldosteronism
Stress*

Renal tubular disorders
Fanconi syndrome
Primary renal glucosuria

Urinary tract haemorrhage with mild hyperglycaemia

Haemoglobin
Haematuria *q.v.*

Haemolysis q.v.
Disseminated intravascular coagulation
Haemoplasmosis
Immune-mediated haemolytic anaemia*
Incompatible blood transfusion
Microangiopathic anaemia
Neonatal isoerythrolysis
Physical causes
- Burns
- Intravenous hypotonic solutions
- Radiation
Splenic torsion
Toxins
- Benzocaine
- Chlorate
- Dimethyl sulphoxide
- Nitrate
- Paracetamol
- Propylthiouracil
- Snake venom

Ketones
Hypoglycaemia, e.g.
- Insulinoma *q.v.*
Low-carbohydrate, high-fat diet
Starvation
Uncontrolled diabetes mellitus/diabetic
ketoacidosis*

Myoglobin – muscle injury/necrosis
Athletic performance
Exercise-induced rhabdomyolysis
Heat stroke*
Ischaemia, e.g.
- Aortic thromboembolism*

Trauma
- Crush injury*

Toxins
- Snakebites

Nitrite

(*Note:* There are many false negatives in dogs and cats.)
  Gram-negative bacteriuria

Protein

False positives (strip test)

Contamination, e.g.
- Benzalkonium chloride
- Cetrimide
- Chlorhexidine

Stale urine

False positives (20% sulphosalicylic acid test)

Cephalosporins
Penicillins
Radiographic contrast media
Sulphafurazole
Thymol
Tolbutamide

Pre-renal

Haemoglobinuria, e.g.
- Haemolytic anaemia*

Hyperproteinaemia *q.v.*

Myoglobinuria, e.g.
- Muscle trauma*
- Rhabdomyolysis

Physiological, e.g.
- Exercise*
- Stress*

Renal

Mild to moderate
- Acute kidney injury *q.v.*
- Amyloidosis

- Breed-associated nephropathy (D)
- Chronic kidney disease* *q.v.*
- Fanconi syndrome
- Glomerulonephritis
- IgA nephropathy
- Primary renal glucosuria
- Secondary glomerular disease
  - Bacterial endocarditis
  - Borreliosis
  - Brucellosis
  - Chronic bacterial infection*
  - Chronic skin disease* *q.v.*
  - Diabetic glomerulosclerosis
  - Dirofilariasis
  - Ehrlichiosis
  - Feline infectious peritonitis* (C)
  - Feline leukaemia virus* (C)
  - Hyperthermia* *q.v.*
  - Hypothermia* *q.v.*
  - Immune-mediated haemolytic anaemia*
  - Infectious canine hepatitis* (D)
  - Inflammatory bowel disease*
  - Leishmaniasis
  - Leptospirosis*
  - Mycoplasma polyarthritis
  - Pancreatitis*
  - Polyarthritis
  - Prostatitis*
  - Pyometra*
  - Pyrexia* *q.v.*
  - Rocky Mountain spotted fever (D)
  - Septicaemia*
  - Sulphonamide hypersensitivity
  - Systemic lupus erythematosus

Severe
- Amyloidosis
- Glomerulonephritis

Post-renal
  Genital tract inflammation
  - Prostatitis*
  - Vaginitis*
  Genital tract secretions
  Urinary tract inflammation
  - Trauma*
  - Urinary tract infection*
  - Urolithiasis*
  Urogenital neoplasia
  - Bladder neoplasia
  - Ureteral neoplasia
  - Urethral neoplasia
  - Vaginal or prostatic neoplasia

pH

DECREASED (<7)
  Acidifying diets*
  Drugs
  - Ammonium chloride
  - Frusemide
  - Methionine
  - Sodium acid phosphate
  - Sodium chloride
  Metabolic acidosis* *q.v.*
  Respiratory acidosis* *q.v.*

INCREASED
  Artefact
  - Contamination with ammonia and detergents
  - Old sample
  Diet
  - Low protein*
  - Postprandial alkaline tide*
  Drugs
  - Acetazolamide
  - Chlorothiazides
  - Potassium citrate

- Sodium bicarbonate
- Sodium lactate

Metabolic alkalosis *q.v.*

Urinary tract disease

- Proximal renal tubular acidosis
- Urinary retention*
- Urinary tract infection with urea-producing bacteria*

Urobilinogen

(*Note:* Of limited use in veterinary medicine)

Re-establishment of bile flow after an episode of biliary obstruction

4.4.3   Abnormalities in urine sediment

Casts

Bilirubin

- Bilirubinuria

Broad casts

- Chronic pyelonephritis
- Dilated renal tubules

Epithelial cell, fatty, granular and waxy casts

- Acute kidney injury *q.v.*
- Chronic kidney disease* *q.v.*
- Degeneration/necrosis of tubular epithelial cells
- Degeneration of white cells
- Glomerulopathy

Haemoglobin

- Haemoglobinuria *q.v.*

Hyaline

- Associated with proteinuria *q.v.*

Myoglobin

- Myoglobinuria *q.v.*

Red blood cell

- Renal tubular haemorrhage

White cell

- Tubulointerstitial inflammation

Crystals (predisposing factors)

Bilirubin

(See Bilirubinuria and Hyperbilirubinaemia)

Calcium oxalate

Diet

- Excess calcium
- Excess oxalic acid
- Excess vitamin C
- Excess vitamin D

Ethylene glycol poisoning

Hyperadrenocorticism

Hypercalciuria

- Hypercalcaemia *q.v.*

Calcium phosphate

Alkaline urine

Primary hyperparathyroidism

Renal tubular acidosis

Cystine

Acid pH

Inherited defect of renal
tubular cells

Silica

Dietary

- Gluten
- Soya bean hulls

Soil ingestion

Struvite

Alkaline urine*

Urinary bladder foreign body

Urinary tract infection*

Urate

Acid urine

Breed associated

- Dalmatian*
- English bulldog

Portosystemic shunts

Urinary tract infection*

Xanthine
Allopurinol administration
Hereditary

Increased red blood cells
Haematuria *q.v.*

Increased white blood cells
Low numbers – normal
Neoplasia
Urinary tract infection*
Urinary tract inflammation*
Urolithiasis*

4.4.4   Infectious agents

Bacteria
Contamination*
- Catheterised sample*
- Failure of sterile collection technique
- Voided sample*

Urinary tract infection*

Fungi
Blastomycosis
Candidiasis
Contaminants*
Cryptococcosis
Prolonged antibiotic therapy

Parasites
Capillaria ova
Dioctophyma renale ova
Dirofilaria microfilaria
Faecal contamination*

Predisposing factors to urinary tract infection

Alteration of urothelium
Changes in normal flora of distal urogenital tract

Drugs
- Cyclophosphamide
- Oestrogens

Metaplasia
- Oestrogens
  - Exogenous
  - Sertoli cell tumours*

Neoplasia*

Trauma
- External*
- Iatrogenic, e.g.
  - Catheterisation*
  - Palpation
  - Surgery*
- Urolithiasis*

Alterations in urine

Decreased frequency of urination
- Involuntary retention*
- Voluntary retention*

Decreased volume
- Decreased water consumption*
- Increased fluid loss*
- Oliguric/anuric kidney injury *q.v.*

Dilute urine*

Glucosuria*

Anatomic defects

Acquired
- Chronic lower urinary tract disease*
- Secondary vesicoureteral reflux
- Surgical procedures

Congenital
- Ectopic ureters
- Persistent urachal diverticula
- Primary vesicoureteral reflux
- Urethral

Immunodeficiency

Congenital diseases

Hyperadrenocorticism
Iatrogenic, e.g.
- Corticosteroids*
Uraemia* *q.v.*

Interference with normal micturition
Outflow obstruction
- Neoplasia*
- Prostatic disease*
- Strictures
- Urinary bladder herniation
- Urolithiasis*
Incomplete emptying of bladder
- Anatomic defects
  - Diverticula
  - Vesicoureteral reflux
- Neurogenic
  - Reflex dyssynergia*
  - Spinal disease

4.5   Cytological findings

4.5.1   Tracheal/bronchoalveolar lavage

Increased neutrophils
Aspiration pneumonia*
Bacterial bronchitis*
Bronchopneumonia*
Canine tracheobronchitis* (D)
Chronic bronchitis*
Foreign body*
Parasites, e.g.
- *Angiostrongylus vasorum*

Increased eosinophils
Drugs
- Potassium bromide (C)
Eosinophilic bronchitis*

Feline asthma* (C)
Parasites
- *Aelurostrongylus abstrusus*
- *Angiostrongylus vasorum*
- *Capillaria aerophila*
- *Crenosoma vulpis*
- *Oslerus* spp.

Pulmonary infiltrate with eosinophils/eosinophilic
bronchopneumopathy

Organisms visible on microscopy/detectable on culture

Upper respiratory tract
Aelurostrongylus abstrusus
Bordetella bronchiseptica
Capillaria aerophila
Malassezia pachydermatis
Mycobacteria spp.
Mycoplasma spp.
Oslerus osleri

Lower respiratory tract
Aelurostrongylus abstrusus
Aspergillus spp.
Blastomyces dermatitidis
*Bordetella bronchiseptica**
Capillaria aerophila
Coccidioides immitis
Crenosoma vulpis (D)
Cryptococcus neoformans
Eucoleus aerophilus
Haemophilus felis
Histoplasma capsulatum
Mycobacteria spp.
Mycoplasma spp.
Opportunistic bacteria*
- *Pasteurella* spp.
- *Pseudomonas* spp.
- *Salmonella* Typhimurium
Oslerus spp.

Paragonimus kellicotti (D)
Penicillium spp.
Pneumocystis carinii (D)
Toxocara canis
Toxoplasma gondii
Yersinia pestis

4.5.2 Nasal flush cytology

Inflammation

Acute or chronic inflammation secondary to foreign body or dental disease*
Allergic rhinitis*
Granulomatous rhinitis
Lymphoplasmacytic rhinitis*
Nasopharyngeal polyp*
Oronasal fistula

Neoplasia

Adenocarcinoma*
Chondrosarcoma
Esthesioneuroblastoma
Fibrosarcoma
Haemangiosarcoma
Histiocytoma
Leiomyosarcoma
Liposarcoma
Lymphoma*
Malignant fibrous histiocytoma
Malignant melanoma
Malignant nerve sheath tumour
Mast cell tumour
Myxosarcoma
Neuroendocrine tumour
Osteosarcoma
Paranasal meningioma
Rhabdomyosarcoma
Squamous cell carcinoma*
Transitional cell carcinoma

Transmissible venereal tumour
Undifferentiated carcinoma*
Undifferentiated sarcoma

Organisms visible on microscopy/detectable on culture

Bacterial/mycoplasmal disease
  Bordetella bronchiseptica*
  Chlamydophila felis* (C)
  Haemophilus felis
  Mycoplasma spp.*

Fungal disease
  Aspergillosis
  Cryptococcosis
  Penicillium spp.
  Rhinosporidium spp.

Parasites
  Capillaria aerophila
  Cuterebra spp.
  Eucoleus böehmi
  Linguatula serrata
  Pneumonyssoides caninum (D)

4.5.3 Liver cytology

Note that cytology of the liver often has low diagnostic value.

Amyloidosis
Hyperplasia
  Nodular hyperplasia*

Increased bile pigment
  Cholestasis* *q.v.*

Increased copper
  Copper-associated hepatopathy

Infectious hepatopathies
  Babesiosis
  Bacillus piliformis

Bacterial cholangiohepatitis*
Canine adenovirus-1* (D)
Canine herpesvirus (D)
Capillaria hepatica
Cytauxzoonosis
Ehrlichiosis
Extrahepatic sepsis
Feline coronavirus* (C)
Hepatozoon canis
Leishmaniasis
Leptospirosis*
Liver abscess
Metorchis conjunctus
Mycobacteriosis
Neosporosis
Opisthorchis felineus
Rhodococcus equi
Toxoplasmosis
Yersiniosis

Inflammatory hepatopathies

Cholangiohepatitis* *q.v.*
Chronic hepatitis* *q.v.*
Copper retention/storage disease
Drugs
- Anticonvulsants
- NSAIDs
Granulomatous hepatitis
- *Bartonella henselae*
- Fungal disease
- Intestinal lymphangitis/lymphangiectasia
- Leishmaniasis
Idiosyncratic drug reaction
Lobular dissecting hepatitis

Neoplastic cells, e.g.

Bile duct carcinoma
Haemangiosarcoma
Hepatocellular adenocarcinoma*
Leiomyosarcoma

Lymphoma*
Mast cell
Metastatic tumour*

Vacuolar hepatopathies

Chronic infections, e.g.
- Dental disease*
- Pyelonephritis

Diabetes mellitus*
Exogenous glucocorticoid administration*
Hyperadrenocorticism
Hyperlipidaemia
Hypothyroidism* (D)
Inflammatory bowel disease*
Lipid storage disease
Neoplasia*
Pancreatitis*

4.5.4 Kidney cytology

Note that cytology of the kidney often has low diagnostic value.

Inflammatory cells

Chronic interstitial nephritis*
Glomerulonephritis
Leptospirosis*
Neoplasia
Pyelonephritis
Renal abscess

Neoplastic cells

Adenocarcinoma
Chondrosarcoma
Haemangioma
Haemangiosarcoma
Lymphoma*
Metastatic thyroid adenocarcinoma
Osteosarcoma

4.5.5 Skin scrapes/hair plucks/tape impressions

Fungi
Dermatophytosis
Malassezia spp.

Parasites
Cheyletiella spp.*
Demodex spp.*
Felicola subrostratus
Heterodoxus spiniger
Larval ticks
Linognathus setosus
Lynxacarus radovskyi
Notoedres cati
*Otodectes cynotis**
*Sarcoptes scabiei** (D)
Trichodectes canis
Trombiculid mites*

4.5.6 Cerebrospinal fluid (CSF) analysis

RAISED CSF WHITE CELL COUNT AND/OR PROTEIN LEVELS

Infectious

Algal
Protothecosis

Bacterial
Leptospirosis
Various aerobes and anaerobes, e.g.
- *Escherichia coli*
- *Klebsiella* spp.
- *Streptococcus* spp.

Fungal
Aspergillosis
Blastomycosis
Coccidioidomycosis
Cryptococcosis
Histoplasmosis
Hyalohyphomycosis
Phaeohyphomycosis

Parasitic
Ancylostoma caninum
Angiostrongylus cantonensis
Cuterebra spp.
Dirofilaria immitis
Toxocara canis

Protozoal
Acanthamoebiasis
Babesiosis
Encephalitozoonosis
Neosporosis
Sarcocystis-like organism
Toxoplasmosis
Trypanosomiasis

Rickettsial
Ehrlichiosis
Rocky Mountain spotted fever (D)
Salmon poisoning disease (D)

Viral
Borna disease virus
Canine distemper* (D)
Canine herpesvirus (D)
Canine parainfluenza (D)
Canine parvovirus* (D)
Central European tick-borne encephalitis
Feline immunodeficiency virus* (C)
Feline infectious peritonitis* (C)

Feline leukaemia virus* (C)
Infectious canine hepatitis* (D)
Pseudorabies
Rabies

Non-infectious
Eosinophilic meningoencephalitis
Fibrocartilaginous embolism
Fucosidosis
Globoid cell leukodystrophy
Granulomatous meningoencephalomyelitis
Idiopathic tremor syndrome
Intervertebral disc disease
Meningoencephalomyelitis in pointers
Necrotising encephalitis
Neoplasia
Periventricular encephalitis
Polioencephalomyelitis
Pug and Maltese encephalitis
Pyogranulomatous meningoencephalomyelitis
Steroid-responsive meningoencephalomyelitis and polyarteritis
Yorkshire terrier encephalitis

4.5.7 Fine-needle aspiration of cutaneous/ subcutaneous masses

Neoplasia

Epithelial
Basal cell tumour
Papilloma
Perianal adenoma*
Sebaceous adenoma/hyperplasia*
Sebaceous gland tumours*
Squamous cell carcinoma*
Sweat gland tumours

Mesenchymal
Haemangiopericytoma
Lipoma*

Sarcoma*, e.g.
- Chondrosarcoma
- Fibrosarcoma
- Haemangiosarcoma
- Osteosarcoma

Round cell
Histiocytoma* (D)
Lymphoma
Mast cell tumour*
Melanoma
Plasmacytoma
- Transmissible venereal tumour (D)

Inflammatory cells
Abscess*
Cellulitis*
Panniculitis
Pyoderma*

4.6 Hormones/endocrine testing

4.6.1 Thyroxine

Decreased
Neonatal cats*
Normal value is lower in sighthounds

Drugs
Amiodarone
Anabolic steroids
Anaesthetics
Anticonvulsants
- Phenobarbitone
- Phenytoin
Frusemide
Glucocorticoids
Iodine supplementation

Methimazole
NSAIDs
- Carprofen
- Flunixin
- Phenylbutazone
- Salicylates

Progestagens
Propranolol
Propylthiouracil
Sulphonamides

Non-thyroidal illness (sick euthyroid syndrome)*, many conditions, e.g.
Acute diseases
- Acute hepatitis* *q.v.*
- Acute pancreatitis*
- Acute kidney injury *q.v.*
- Autoimmune haemolytic anaemia*
- Bacterial bronchopneumonia*
- Canine distemper virus* (D)
- Intervertebral disc disease* (D)
- Polyradiculoneuritis
- Sepsis*
- Systemic lupus erythematosus

Chronic diseases
- Cachexia
  - Cardiac*
  - Neoplasia*
- Chronic kidney disease* *q.v.*
- Congestive heart failure*
- Dermatological disease* *q.v.*
- Diabetes mellitus*
- Gastrointestinal disease* *q.v.*
- Hyperadrenocorticism
- Hypoadrenocorticism (D)
- Liver disease* *q.v.*
- Lymphoma*
- Megaoesophagus
- Systemic mycoses

Primary hypothyroidism
  Acquired*
  Congenital

Increased
  - Diet
  - Soy

Hyperthyroidism* (C)
Juvenile dogs*
Obesity*
Pregnant bitches*
Strenuous exercise*
Total T4 autoantibodies
Thyroid carcinoma
Drugs
  - Excessive thyroid hormone supplementation
  - Ipodate

4.6.2 Parathyroid hormone

Decreased
  Artefact
  - Prolonged storage/transport above freezing

  Hypervitaminosis D
  Non-parathyroid causes of hypercalcaemia
  Primary hypoparathyroidism
  Drugs that increase serum calcium
  (see Hypercalcaemia)

Increased
  Hyperadrenocorticism
  Non-parathyroid causes of hypocalcaemia *q.v.*
  Nutritional secondary hyperparathyroidism
  Primary hyperparathyroidism
  Renal secondary hyperparathyroidism*
  Drugs that decrease serum calcium
  (see Hypocalcaemia)

4.6.3 Cortisol (baseline or post-ACTH stimulation test)

Increased
Severe/chronic illness*
Stress*

Artefact
Cross-reaction with glucocorticoids
(but not dexamethasone)
- Cortisone
- Hydrocortisone
- Methylprednisolone
- Prednisolone
- Prednisone

Drugs
Anticonvulsants

Hyperadrenocorticism
Adrenal dependent
Pituitary dependent

Decreased

Artefact
Prolonged/improper storage of ACTH
Incorrect administration of ACTH

Drugs
Chronic androgen administration
Chronic glucocorticoid administration
Chronic progestagen administration
Megestrol acetate

Hypoadrenocorticism (D)
Primary
Secondary

4.6.4 Insulin

With concurrent hyperglycaemia

Decreased
Diabetes mellitus*

Increased
Insulin-binding antibodies
Insulin resistance*
With concurrent hypoglycaemia

Increased
Insulinoma

4.6.5 ACTH

Decreased
Adrenal-dependent hyperadrenocorticism
Iatrogenic hyperadrenocorticism
Spontaneous secondary hyperadrenocorticism

Artefact
Collecting into glass containers
Storing above freezing

Increased
Ectopic ACTH secretion
Insulin administration
Pituitary-dependent hyperadrenocorticism
Primary hypoadrenocorticism

4.6.6 Vitamin D (1,25-dihydroxycholecalciferol)

Decreased
Chronic kidney disease
Lymphoma

Primary hyperparathyroidism
Vitamin D-deficient diet

Increased

Exogenous administration
Granulomatous disease
Humoral hypercalcaemia of malignancy
Primary hyperparathyroidism
Vitamin D-based rodenticides

4.6.7 Testosterone

Decreased

Castrated male
Sertoli cell tumour*
Drugs
* Exogenous androgen treatment

Artefact

Collection into EDTA
Storage at room temperature
Storage with red blood cells

Increased (post GnRH or hCG)

Functional testicular tissue
Ovarian thecoma

4.6.8 Progesterone

Decreased

Artefact
* Storage at room temperature
* Storage in whole blood
Exogenous progestagen administration
Failure to maintain normal luteal function
Failure to ovulate

Imminent parturition
Normal anoestrus

Increased

Adrenocortical carcinoma
Granulosa cell tumour
Luteal cysts
Normal luteal function
Ovarian remnant syndrome
Prostaglandin therapy
Recent ovulation

4.6.9   Oestradiol

Increased

Follicular ovarian cysts
Ovarian remnant syndrome
Seminoma*
Sertoli cell tumour*

4.6.10   Pro-BNP

Increased

Acquired cardiac disease, e.g.
- Mitral valve disease *(D)
- Dilated cardiomyopathy *(D)
- Hypertrophic cardiomyopathy *(C)
- Pulmonary hypertension

Congenital cardiac disease, e.g.
- Patent ductus arteriosus

Non-cardiac disease
- Azotaemia
- Babesiosis

Physiological
- Variation over time in an individual

4.7   Faecal analysis findings

4.7.1   Faecal blood

See Haematochezia *q.v.* and Melaena *q.v.*
Note: Tests for occult blood may be positive if red meat has been fed in the previous five days.

4.7.2   Faecal parasites

Cardiorespiratory parasites shed in faeces

Aelurostrongylus abstrusus
Angiostrongylus
Capillaria aerophila
Crenosoma vulpis (D)
Eucoleus boehmi
Paragonimus kellicotti (D)

Flukes

Alaria spp.

Hookworms

Ancylostoma* spp.
Uncinaria* spp.

Protozoa

Cryptosporidium* spp.
Giardia* spp.
Toxoplasma gondii
Tritrichomonas foetus

Roundworms

Toxascaris leonina
Toxocara canis
Toxocara cati

Tapeworms

Taenia* spp.

Threadworm
Strongyloides spp.

Whipworms
Trichuris vulpis *

4.7.3 Faecal culture

Culture for specific enteropathogenic bacteria
Campylobacter spp. *
Clostridium difficile *
Clostridium perfringens *
Escherichia coli *
- Enterohaemorrhagic
- Enteropathogenic
- Enterotoxigenic

Salmonella spp. *
Yersinia spp.

Non-selective culture
Non-selective culture is thought to be of limited diagnostic use.

4.7.4 Faecal fungal infections

Histoplasma capsulatum

4.7.5 Undigested food residues

Note: Trypsinogen-like immunoreactivity is a more sensitive test for exocrine pancreatic insufficiency than is the presence of undigested food residues.

Fat
Bile acid deficiency
Exocrine pancreatic insufficiency
Malabsorption*

Starch
Exocrine pancreatic insufficiency
High-starch diet
Increased intestinal transit time

PART 5
ELECTRODIAGNOSTIC TESTING

5.1 Electrocardiographic findings

Note: Changes in ECG measurements are relatively insensitive indicators of chamber size.

5.1.1 Alterations in P wave

Tall P wave (P pulmonale)
Right atrial enlargement, e.g.
- Chronic respiratory disease*
- Dilated cardiomyopathy*
- Tricuspid regurgitation*

Wide P wave (P mitrale)
Left atrial enlargement*, e.g.
- Dilated cardiomyopathy*
- Mitral regurgitation*

Variable height of P wave (wandering pacemaker)
Increased vagal tone*

Differential Diagnosis in Small Animal Medicine, Second Edition.
Alex Gough and Kate Murphy.
© 2015 John Wiley & Sons, Ltd. Published 2015 by John Wiley & Sons, Ltd.

Absent P wave

Atrial fibrillation*
Acute atrial stretch
  • Volume overload
Atrial pathology
Excessive vagal stimulation
Large atria*

Persistent atrial standstill
Artefact
Atrial pathology
Hyperkalaemia

Sinus arrest/sino-atrial block
Normal in brachycephalics
Drugs, e.g.
  • Beta blockers
  • Calcium channel blockers
  • Digitalis glycosides
Atrial disease, e.g.
  • Cardiomyopathy*
  • Dilatation*
  • Fibrosis
  • Hypertrophy
  • Necrosis
Electrolyte imbalances*
Increased vagal tone
  • Chronic respiratory disease*
  • Gastrointestinal disease*
Sick sinus syndrome
Stenosis of bundle of His

5.1.2 Alterations in QRS complex

Tall R waves
Left ventricular enlargement, e.g.
  • Cardiomyopathy*
  • Hyperthyroidism* (C)
  • Mitral regurgitation*

Small R waves
Acute haemorrhage
Pericardial effusion

Wide QRS

Supraventricular
Left bundle branch block
- Cardiomyopathy*
- Subaortic stenosis*
- Drugs/toxins, e.g.
  - Doxorubicin
  - Tricyclic antidepressants
Right bundle branch block
- Occasionally seen in normal animals
- Cardiac neoplasia
- Heartworm disease
- Inherited
- Post cardiac arrest
- Ventricular septal defect
Left ventricular hypertrophy*
Microscopic intramural myocardial infarction
Quinidine toxicity
Severe ischaemia

Ventricular
Accelerated idioventricular rhythm*
Ventricular ectopy*
Ventricular escape complexes
Ventricular premature complexes*
Ventricular tachycardia*

Deep S waves
Right ventricular enlargement, e.g.
- Pulmonary hypertension
- Pulmonic stenosis
- Reverse-shunting patent ductus arteriosus
- Tricuspid regurgitation

Electrical alternans
Pericardial effusion

Slurred upstroke

Ventricular pre-excitation/Wolff–Parkinson–White syndrome
- Acquired heart defects, e.g.
- Feline hypertrophic cardiomyopathy
- Congenital
- Idiopathic

5.1.3 Alterations in P–R relationship

Prolonged P–R interval (first-degree atrioventricular block)

Occasionally seen in normal animals*
Age-related degeneration of atrioventricular conduction system
Drugs/toxins
- Beta blockers
- Calcium channel blockers
- Cardiac glycosides
- Quinidine
- Tricyclic antidepressants
- Vitamin D rodenticides

Feline dilated cardiomyopathy (C)
Heart disease*
Hyperkalaemia *q.v.*
Hypokalaemia* *q.v.*
Increased vagal tone*

Short P–R interval

Ventricular pre-excitation/Wolff–Parkinson–White syndrome
- Acquired heart defects, e.g.
- Feline hypertrophic cardiomyopathy
- Congenital
- Idiopathic

Intermittent failure of atrioventricular conduction (second-degree atrioventricular block)

May be seen in normal animals
Juvenile puppies at rest
Physiological when seen associated with supraventricular tachycardia

Drugs, e.g.
- Alpha-2 agonists
- Atropine
- Beta blockers
- Calcium channel blockers
- Cardiac glycosides

Electrolyte imbalances* *q.v.*, e.g.
- Hyperkalaemia *q.v.*

Hyperthyroidism* (C)

Increased vagal tone, e.g.
- Chronic respiratory disease* *q.v.*
- Gastrointestinal disease* *q.v.*

Microscopic idiopathic fibrosis
Myocardial diseases
Stenosis of bundle of His

Complete atrioventricular block (third-degree atrioventricular block)

Idiopathic
Bacterial endocarditis
Congenital heart defects, e.g.
- Aortic stenosis
- Ventricular septal defect

Hyperkalaemia
Isolated congenital atrioventricular block
Myocardial diseases including infiltrative disorders
Myocardial infarction
Myocarditis
Severe drug intoxication, e.g.
- Beta blockers
- Calcium channel blockers
- Cardiac glycosides

5.1.4   Alterations in S–T segment

S–T segment depression/slur

Acute myocardial infarction
Cardiac trauma
Digitalis toxicity

Electrolyte disturbances* *q.v.*
Myocardial ischaemia

S–T segment elevation
Myocardial hypoxia
Myocardial infarction
Myocardial neoplasia
Pericarditis

Secondary changes to S–T segment following QRS abnormalities
Bundle branch block
Ventricular hypertrophy
Ventricular premature complexes*

Pseudo-depression of S–T segment (prominent atrial repolarisation wave)
Pathological atrial changes
Tachycardia *q.v.*

5.1.5 Alterations in Q–T interval

Prolonged Q–T interval
Central nervous system disease *q.v.*
Drugs/toxins
- Amiodarone
- Ethylene glycol
- Quinidine
- Tick paralysis
- Tricyclic antidepressants

Exercise*
Hypocalcaemia *q.v.*
Hypokalaemia* *q.v.*
Hypothermia* *q.v.*

Shortened Q–T interval
Hypercalcaemia *q.v.*
Hyperkalaemia *q.v.*
Drugs/toxins
- Cardiac glycosides

5.1.6   Alterations in T wave

Tall T waves

Anaesthetic complications
Bradycardia *q.v.*
Heart failure*
Hyperkalaemia *q.v.*
Hyperventilation during heat stroke
Left bundle branch block
Myocardial hypoxia
Myocardial infarction
Right bundle branch block

Small T waves

Hypokalaemia* *q.v.*

T wave alternans

Hypocalcaemia *q.v.*
Increased circulating catecholamines
Increased sympathetic tone

5.1.7   Alterations in baseline

Atrial fibrillation
Atrial flutter
Movement artefact*
Ventricular fibrillation
Ventricular flutter

5.1.8   Rhythm alterations

Atrial fibrillation

Anaesthesia
Gastrointestinal disease*
Hypoadrenocorticism (D)
Hypothyroidism* (D)
Primary/'lone'

Rapid, large-volume pericardiocentesis
Severe atrial enlargement, e.g.
- Dilated cardiomyopathy*
- Mitral regurgitation*
- Patent ductus arteriosus
Volume overload

Atrial flutter

Cardiomyopathy
Iatrogenic
- Cardiac catheterisation
Severe atrial enlargement, e.g.
- Dilated cardiomyopathy*
- Mitral regurgitation*
- Patent ductus arteriosus
Drugs
- Quinidine

Atrioventricular block q.v.

Parasystole

Atrial
Ventricular

Persistent atrial standstill

Artefact
Atrial pathology
Hyperkalaemia

Sinus block/arrest

Atrial disease, e.g.
- Cardiomyopathy*
- Dilatation*
- Fibrosis
- Hypertrophy
- Necrosis
Electrolyte imbalances* q.v.
Increased vagal tone
- Chronic respiratory disease*
- Gastrointestinal disease*
Sick sinus syndrome

Stenosis of bundle of His
Drugs, e.g.
- Beta blockers
- Calcium channel blockers
- Digitalis glycosides

Supraventricular premature complexes/ supraventricular tachycardia (sinus, atrial or junctional tachycardia)

May be normal

Structural cardiac disease, e.g.
Atrial enlargement*
Myocardial disease

Systemic disease, e.g.
Drugs, e.g.
- Digoxin
- General anaesthesia
Hyperthyroidism* (C)
Inflammation*
Neoplasia*
Sepsis*

Ventricular premature complexes/ventricular tachycardia

Cardiac disease
Cardiomyopathy, e.g. dilated cardiomyopathy and arrhythmogenic right ventricular cardiomyopathy
Congestive heart failure*
Endocarditis, e.g.
- Bacterial
Inherited, e.g.
- German Shepherd dogs
Myocardial infarction
Myocarditis, e.g.
- Idiopathic
- Traumatic
- Viral

Neoplasia
Pericarditis

Extra-cardiac disease
Anaemia* *q.v.*
Autonomic imbalances*
Coagulopathies *q.v.*
Disseminated intravascular
coagulation
Drugs/toxins
- Atropine
- Anti-dysrhythmics, e.g.
  - Amiodarone
  - Digoxin
  - Lignocaine
  - Sotalol
- Dobutamine
- Dopamine
- Glycopyrronium bromide
- Halothane
- Propantheline bromide
- Theobromine
- Tricyclic antidepressants
- Xylazine
- Vitamin D rodenticides
Endocrinopathies*
Gastric dilatation/volvulus*
Hypoxia
Nutritional deficiencies
Pancreatitis*
Sepsis*
Uraemia* *q.v.*

Ventricular flutter/fibrillation

Ventricular asystole

Electrolyte/acid–base disorders
Severe sino-atrial block

Terminal systemic disease
Third-degree atrioventricular block

5.1.9 Alterations in rate

Tachycardia

Sinus tachycardia
Physiological
- Excitement*
- Exercise*
- Fear*
- Pain*

Drugs/toxins
- Adder bites
- Baclofen
- Blue-green algae
- Cannabis
- Ethylene glycol
- Glyphosate
- Ibuprofen
- Metaldehyde
- Paracetamol
- Paraquat
- Petroleum distillates
- Phenoxy acid herbicides
- Pyrethrins/pyrethroids
- Salbutamol
- Selective serotonin reuptake inhibitors
- Terfenadine
- Theobromine
- Tricyclic antidepressants
- Vitamin D rodenticides
- Heart failure*
- Respiratory disease*
- Shock*

Pathological
- Systemic disease
  - Anaemia* *q.v.*
  - Fever* *q.v.*

- Hyperthyroidism* (C)
- Hypoxia
- Sepsis*

Other supraventricular tachycardia
Atrial fibrillation
Atrial flutter
Ectopic atrial tachycardia
Junctional tachycardia
- Automatic junctional tachycardia
- AV nodal re-entrant tachycardia
- Bypass tract-mediated macro-re-entrant tachycardia
Sinus nodal re-entrant tachycardia
Ventricular pre-excitation/Wolff–Parkinson–White syndrome
Ventricular tachycardia *q.v.*

Bradycardia
Atrial standstill
- Atrioventricular myopathy
- Dilated cardiomyopathy*
- Hyperkalaemia *q.v.*
Heart block *q.v.*
Sick sinus syndrome
Sinus arrest

Sinus bradycardia
Normal in athletic dogs, during
rest/sleep
Cardiac disease
- End-stage heart failure*
- Feline dilated cardiomyopathy (C)
Drugs/toxins
- Adder bites
Anti-dysrhythmics
- Beta blockers
- Calcium channel blockers
- Digoxin
- Baclofen
- Cannabis

- Carbamate
- Daffodil
- Glyphosate
- Ivermectin
- Loperamide
- Organophosphates
- Paraquat
- Phenoxy acid herbicides
- Rhododendron
- Theobromine
- Vitamin D rodenticides
- Yew

Hypoglycaemia *q.v.*
Hypothyroidism*
Increased vagal tone, e.g.
- Gastrointestinal disease* *q.v.*
- Respiratory disease* *q.v.*

Neurological disease, e.g.
- Coma

Severe systemic disease*

5.2 Electromyographic findings

5.2.1 Spontaneous activity

Normal end-plate noise
Electrode-insertion artefact
Fibrillation potentials
- Denervation

Myotonic potentials
(dive bomber sound)
- Myotonia

Pseudo-myotonic potentials
- Polymyositis
- Primary myopathies
- Steroid myopathy

5.2.2 Evoked activity

Decreased muscle action potential
Junctionopathies
- Botulism
- Tick paralysis

Neuropathies
Primary myopathies

Increased muscle action potential
Aged animals
Chronic neuropathies

Decremental decrease after repeated stimulation
Myasthenia gravis
Re-innervation

5.3 Nerve conduction velocity findings

5.3.1 Decreased velocity

Demyelinating neuropathies
Distal part of extremity
Hypothermia of adjacent tissues*
Protein malnutrition
Very old/young animals*

5.3.2 Increased velocity

Proximal part of extremity

Index

Differential Diagnosis in Small Animal Medicine, Second Edition.
Alex Gough and Kate Murphy.
© 2015 John Wiley & Sons, Ltd. Published 2015 by John Wiley & Sons, Ltd.